Mental Illness in Children

Special Issue Editor
Rosemary Sheehan

MDPI • Basel • Beijing • Wuhan • Barcelona • Belgrade

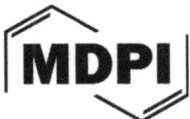

MDPI

Special Issue Editor
Rosemary Sheehan
Monash University
Australia

Editorial Office
MDPI
St. Alban-Anlage 66
Basel, Switzerland

This edition is a reprint of the Special Issue published online in the open access journal *Brain Sciences* (ISSN 2076-3425) in 2017 (available at: http://www.mdpi.com/journal/brainsci/special_issues/ mental_illness_children).

For citation purposes, cite each article independently as indicated on the article page online and as indicated below:

Lastname, F.M.; Lastname, F.M. Article title. *Journal Name* **Year**, *Article number*, page range.

First Edition 2018

ISBN 978-3-03842-881-7 (Pbk)
ISBN 978-3-03842-882-4 (PDF)

Table of Contents

About the Special Issue Editor

Rosemary Sheehan teaches mental health in the postgraduate social work programme and is Director of the Higher Degrees by Research programme. Her published research covers a range of areas: child welfare and the law, family violence, mental health, judicial and corrections responses to offenders, with particular reference to women offenders, and social work curricula. Her recent publications include: Working within the Forensic Paradigm: Cross-discipline approaches for policy and practice (with James Ogloff. Routledge, 2015); Australia's Children's Courts Today and Tomorrow (with Allan Borowski) (2013, Springer); Children and the Law: International Approaches to Children and their Vulnerabilities, (with Helen Rhoades and Nicky Stanley. Jessica Kingsley, 2012); studies which examine child wellbeing and vulnerability within the welfare jurisdiction. Professor Sheehan has 17 years' experience conducting alternative dispute resolution conferences at the Children's Court, Victoria, Australia. Her current research projects include: child protection and legal responses to cumulative harm in children (Victorian Government funded) and the cross-over between youth offending and child protection in children and young people before the Children's Court, Victoria (Federal Government funded).

Preface to "Mental Illness in Children"

1. Childhood Development: Life Stages and Their Impact

Childhood is a stage of life that is filled with potential for development, and the early years of childhood see immense physical changes in growth; mastery over body functions like movement; the acquisition of language and cognitive development to understand their own and others' thinking and reasoning; and the psychosocial development of trust in the world, comfort in the care they receive from parents and caregivers, and the sense of being secure in themselves that this engenders. Bowlby placed great emphasis on the enduring emotional bonds the child needs to develop with key adults in their early life, identifying security and healthy family processes as important factors in future resilience and social competence [1]. This human development approach to child growth and development identifies what a child needs at any particular age to promote normal growth and development, to minimise risk, and foster protective factors to ensure that they thrive and prosper.

The concepts of 'normative' or 'non-normative' development are often applied to gain a sense of whether or not a child is in a 'healthy or desirable state for someone to be in at a given age' ([2], p. 109). When something is characterised as non-normative, it suggests that what is happening is not usual or typical, with perhaps gaps in a child's individual functioning resulting in some subsequent impairment. When health is impaired, it can have minor to major impacts on a child's emotional and social wellbeing.

A child's health status is also influenced by parental factors, such as a family's socioeconomic situation. Poverty and low family income can adversely affect the health, education, and self-esteem of children, compromising their growth and development and general societal participation. A parent's own ill-health, mental illness, housing instability, or social isolation can affect their capacity to effectively parent their child, provide them with supportive childhood relationships, and ensure their access to the services they need to protect them from the development of health problems. The impact of chronic stress on a child and how this can affect their development is well noted [3].

2. The Impact of Mental Health Problems

The prevalence of mental disorder in children in Australia finds that around one in seven (13.9%) children and adolescents aged 4–17 years, experience a mental disorder [4], equivalent to an estimated 560,000 Australian children and adolescents. Many of these children and young people are not in contact with therapeutic or support services, their mental distress left unacknowledged and without intervention, with increased risk of growing and developing with personal and social difficulties. These difficulties are frequently associated with challenges across family, education and learning, school attendance, physical health, and offending behaviour [5]. The primary health care system is typically the 'front door' for children with mental health concerns, with the specialist Child and Adolescent Mental Health Services offering a service for children with more severe problems. However, access to these services can be difficult, with lengthy waiting times, the need to prove eligibility for a service, and the often short-term service responses, all of which increase vulnerability and can have a devastating impact on family life [6].

By and large, the mental health problems children experience can be categorised as behaviour disorders, developmental disorders, and emotional disorders [6]. Behaviour (or conduct) disorders are characterised by a pattern of antisocial, aggressive, or deviant behaviour. The DSM-5 (Diagnostic and Statistical Manual of Mental Disorders) [4] states that children exhibiting these behaviours, which are more than 'childish mischief or adolescent rebelliousness' ([6], p. 80), are hostile or defiant in their interactions with others and may show little remorse for their behaviour. These behaviours are influenced by environment, family, and child-specific factors, such as a 'difficult' temperament, brain injury, chronic illness, or cognitive deficits ([6], p. 81). Attention deficit hyperactivity disorder has been a prominent explanation assigned to children who are highly distractible, hyperactive, and impulsive, and there has been controversy about its diagnostic application and reliance on drugs as an intervention. Certainly, however, there are considerable negative consequences for children who are unable to achieve at school, whose learning is significantly impaired, and whose behaviours impair their social interactions.

Autism and Asperger's syndrome (autism spectrum disorders) are the developmental disorders most identified in children. Autism commences before three years of age and is thought to have an organic, brain development basis. Children with autism struggle with physical contact, avoid eye contact, have speech and language disorders, do not cope with changes in their environment, and engage in repetitive behaviours. Children with Asperger's syndrome share some features with autism in that they struggle with social interaction and fix on specific interests and behaviours, but they do not have delays in speech and cognitive development. Asperger's syndrome is more commonly associated with boys. As adults, they can function well in employment which calls for detailed and focussed attention, but continue to have social and relational difficulties, compounded by struggling to empathise with the feelings of others. Attention deficit hyperactivity disorder (ADHD) is the most common mental disorder in Australia overall, with the Australian Australian Institute of Health and Welfare (AIHW) (2014) [7] finding that 7.4% of children and adolescents had been assessed as having ADHD in the previous 12 months.

Anxiety disorders were the next most common (6.9%), followed by major depressive disorder (2.8%) and conduct disorder (2.1%). The forms of emotional disorders in children include depression and anxiety, characterised by the same difficulties which beset adults. Childhood depression and anxiety can manifest itself in school refusal, as a consequence of child maltreatment, or behavioural difficulties. Children with major depression have longstanding psychosocial problems, including family conflict, domestic violence, child abuse, school problems such as bullying and isolation, and may also have parents with mental health problems ([6], p. 88). This may be associated with upheaval in a child's life, family distress, or external factors causing distress for the child.

Mental health difficulties for children, if not successfully ameliorated, will continue in their adult lives, albeit often differently expressed. Ongoing conduct disorder is associated with the onset of schizophrenia or sociopathy. Depression and anxiety may remain and be expressed in the range of adult disorders categorised by DSM-5. What is clear is that early intervention into childhood mental health difficulties is imperative, with an integrated service approach, not fragmented and divided as is the current structure throughout much of Australia's mental health services.

3. Supporting the Child and Family

Clinicians typically intervene at times of transition or crisis; primary healthcare, community health centres, hospitals, networks, mental health services, and welfare or government agencies (such as the child protection service) are places where children may seek help for mental health concerns or where their families may come for help with broader family problems which affect a child's mental health and wellbeing.

Working with children in these domains requires specific awareness of how children make sense of mental health problems; what can be expected of them given their age, life, and individual and family circumstances; and what they need from their caregivers for mental health treatment and recovery. The child's dependency on adults to care for and treat them means that clinicians must work as much with family members as with the individual child, in order to meet the child's needs and address stresses as well as ensure that the necessary interventions are put in place. Thus, any assessment of needs must be systemic, always being aware that they must be child-centred, as parental needs and perceptions may differ from what is in the child's best interests. Clinicians in mental health draw not only on theories and knowledge of individual functioning, but also on knowledge of human development, individual and family life stages, and family functioning to effectively and accurately assess the child client's situation.

The scope of intervention in child mental health varies according to the nature of the problem experienced, be it crisis intervention, a chronic mental health condition, or a serious illness. A child may be seen where the presenting problem is not mental health-focused (for example, child abuse and neglect, domestic and family violence), but it is important to keep in mind the child's mental health and assess what impact there is, from the presenting problem, on the child's mental health and wellbeing. It is this person-in-environment perspective of the mental health experience [8] which characterises clinical practice in this domain. For instance, Reference [9] refers to the need to take a holistic approach to understanding people, their problems, and their reactions.

Therapeutic interventions when working with children will, as noted, mostly involve working with the family. Moreover, clinicians must be alert to the range of psychosocial issues which affect recovery and actively work to minimise the consequences of illness and improve health outcomes for the child. We are mindful of factors that can impact the capacity to receive care, and the linkages between 'social illnesses and problems' and mental illness, such as would be seen in child abuse, exemplifying how psychosocial issues will affect a child and their health outcomes ([10], p. 25). Children challenged by mental health problems are particularly vulnerable. In working with children and their families, the occurrence of mental health problems gives primacy to child-centred and strengths-based practice, and exemplifies a systems or holistic approach, as the child is centred in a context of relationships which intersect with both the illness experience and their recovery.

The articles in this special edition canvass a range of issues that intersect with mental illness and children, and offer a variety of experiences by which such illness is understood. The breadth of scholarship herein indicates the many perspectives there are on childhood mental illness, and presents a commendable group of articles to enhance the knowledge and experience of this domain.

Conflicts of Interest: The author declares no conflict of interest.

References

1. Keble-Devlin, B. Disorders of childhood: A developmental and family perspective. In Mental Health in Australia: Collaborative Community Practice, 3rd ed.; Meadows, G., Farhall, J., Fossey, E., Grigg, M., McDermott, F., Singh, B., Eds.; OUP: Melbourne, Australia, 2012; pp. 588–601.
2. Jones, K. Health and Human Behaviour. Oxford Univerity Press: Melbourne, Australia, 2003.
3. Gething, L.; Hatchard, D.; Papalia, D.; Olds, S. Life Span Development; McGraw-Hill: North Ryde, NSW, 1989.
4. American Psychiatric Association. Diagnostic and Statistical Manual of Mental Disorders (DSM-V), 5th ed.; American Psychiatric Association: Washington, DC, USA, 2014.

5. Child and Adolescent Mental Health Service (CAMHS) Review. Children and Young People in Mind: The Final Report of the National CAMHS Review. DoH: London, UK, 2008. Available online: http://webarchive.nationalarchives.gov.uk/20081230004520/publications.dcsf.gov.uk/eorderingdownload/camhs-review.pdf (accessed on 2 August 2017).

6. Gould, N. Mental Health Social Work in Context, 2nd ed.; Routledge: Oxon, UK, 2016.

7. Australian Institute of Health and Welfare (AIHW) (2014). Child health, development and well-being. Available online: http://www.aihw.gov.au/child-health/health/ (accessed on 8 August 2017).

8. Miller, J.; Nilsson, D. Contemporary Issues in Health Social Work. In Social Work: Contexts and Practice, 2nd ed.; Connolly, M., Harms, L., Eds.; OUP: South Melbourne, Australia, 2009.

9. Wodarski, J.; Holosko, M.; Feit, M.D. Evidence-Informed Assessment and Practice in Child Welfare; Springer Publications: New York, NY, USA, 2015.

10. Browne, T.A. Social Work Roles and Health-Care Settings. In Handbook of Health Social Work; Gehlert, S., Browne, T.A., Eds.; John Wiley & Sons, Inc.: Hoboken, NJ, USA, 2006; pp. 23–42.

Rosemary Sheehan
Special Issue Editor

Article

Infants Investigated by the Child Welfare System: Exploring a Distinct Profile of Risks, Service Needs, and Referrals for Support in Ontario

Joanne Filippelli [1,*], Barbara Fallon [1], Esme Fuller-Thomson [1] and Nico Trocmé [2]

1 Factor-Inwentash Faculty of Social Work, University of Toronto, 246 Bloor Street West, Toronto, ON M5S 1V4, Canada; barbara.fallon@utoronto.ca (B.F.); esme.fullerthomson@utoronto.ca (E.F.-T.)
2 Centre for Research on Children and Families, McGill University, 3506 University Street, Montreal, QC H3A 2A7, Canada; nico.trocme@mcgill.ca
* Correspondence: joanne.filippelli@utoronto.ca; Tel.: +1-416-978-1386

Academic Editor: Rosemary Sheehan
Received: 17 July 2017; Accepted: 8 August 2017; Published: 12 August 2017

Abstract: The science of early childhood development underscores that maltreatment and other adversities experienced during infancy heightens the risk for poor developmental and socio-emotional outcomes. Referrals to supportive services by the child welfare system are particularly critical during infancy given the rapidity of brain development and infants' sensitivity to their environment. The main objectives of the current study are to: (1) examine age-specific differences in clinical and case characteristics; (2) determine the factors associated with the service referral decision involving infants; and (3) explore the types of services families have been referred to at the conclusion of a maltreatment-related investigation. Using data from the Ontario Incidence Study of Reported Child Abuse and Neglect for 2013, descriptive analyses were conducted, as was a logistic regression to identify factors associated with the decision to refer families of infants to supportive services. Overall, the findings reveal that the profile of infants and their families differs distinctly from those of older children with respect to risks, service needs, and service referrals, although this is rarely reflected in child welfare practice and policy. Investigations involving infants were most likely to have a referral made to supportive services, least likely to have an infant functioning concern identified; most likely to have a primary caregiver risk factor identified; and, the greatest likelihood of experiencing economic hardship. Multiple risks, identified for the primary caregiver of the infant are correlated to referral decisions for infants. However, the needs of the infant are likely under-identified and require cross-sectorial collaboration.

Keywords: child welfare; infants; referral to services; child maltreatment

1. Introduction

Children and families investigated by the child welfare system often have complex needs that may require various types of supportive services that span across numerous sectors [1–4]. The decision to refer children and families to supportive services can signal the child welfare systems' recognition of child and/or family need [5]. A child welfare worker's decision to refer to services is predicated upon the assessment of need. Identifying child and family needs and aligning services with those needs may help to prevent deterioration in family functioning, decrease the risk of maltreatment and increase the likelihood of family reunification [4,6,7]. Service referrals are an important step in promoting both the safety and well-being of children and can be particularly consequential for infants and young children. Early identification, referral, and intervention may buffer or prevent the developmental consequences of maltreatment and other adversities. Without appropriate intervention, developmental difficulties that emerge in early childhood can become more challenging to address and ameliorate over time [8]. Early identification and intervention are critical as the brain is most receptive to the environment in the first years of life [9]. Yet, there is minimal literature focusing on service referrals within the context of child welfare service provision [10]. There is little understanding of the types of services that children and families are referred to, including referrals to concrete services that may assist families in meeting their basic needs (e.g., food, housing, utilities), educational services (e.g., parent support groups), and clinical services (e.g., mental health counseling) [1,10]. There is no study that has explored the factors associated with the decision to provide service referrals to families of infants; nor, is there a study that has explored the types of services that families of infants and older children are referred to within the context of maltreatment-related investigations in Canada.

1.1. Developmental Issues for Infants

A high rate of developmental concerns has been found in infants and toddlers regardless of whether allegations were substantiated or unsubstantiated [11,12]. Children who remain in the home have shown similar high rates of mental health issues as children placed into out-of-home care [13,14]. For infants and young children involved with the child welfare system, there is a significant gap between the identification of need for mental services and service receipt [14]. Child welfare-involved infants are unlikely to have their developmental and mental health needs met prior to school entry [15]. Infants reported to and investigated by the Ontario child welfare system have been noted to be the least likely group of children to be identified by child welfare workers as having a functioning concern [16]. The lack of identification of developmental issues by the child welfare system can translate into low referral rates to, and underuse of, early intervention services [17,18]. There have been concerns about the adequacy of the child welfare system's response to the unique needs of infants and young children throughout the extant literature [11,18–23].

1.2. Caregiver Concerns

Using the 2008 cycle of the Canadian Incidence Study of Reported Child Abuse and Neglect (CIS-2008), Jud, Fallon, and Trocmé found that caregiver risk factors (e.g., few social supports), younger caregiver age, and socio-economic hardship were significantly associated with the likelihood of receiving ongoing child welfare services or a referral to services post-investigation [24]. Palusci explored post-investigation services and recurrence after confirmed psychological maltreatment for children and found that poverty, drug, or alcohol issues and other forms of violence increased the likelihood of a service referral [25]. Less than one quarter of families were referred to services following confirmed psychological maltreatment.

Caregivers of children involved with the child welfare system have also been noted to experience unmet service needs [26,27]. In Ontario, being a victim of intimate partner violence (IPV), having few social support (i.e., social isolation or lack of social supports), and mental health issues have consistently emerged as the most frequently identified caregiver risk factors in maltreatment-related investigations involving infants [16,28]. Access to social supports from the community can help to buffer stress and reduce social isolation, a risk factor for both infant maltreatment and poor infant psychosocial functioning [29,30]. The importance of social supports in child welfare decision-making is highlighted by research indicating that a caregiver with few social supports is an influential predictor for transferring a case to ongoing child welfare services in two studies exploring maltreatment-related investigations involving infants and their families in Ontario [16,28]. A caregiver's social support network is particularly consequential for infants as it can impact the quality of infant-caregiver relationship [30].

1.3. Factors Associated with Service Referrals and Dispositions

Child welfare workers have been described as service brokers and gateway providers to services for children and youth (e.g., [15,31,32]). A referral made by a child welfare worker for support services is a critical step to match services to needs [33]. The importance of understanding and addressing the needs of infants and young children who come into contact with the child welfare system is underscored by the accumulating evidence of their developmental vulnerabilities, unmet needs, and the underutilization of services [14,15,20]. Research suggests that initial involvement with the child welfare system may increase access to mental health services [15].

Despite the consequential nature of the service referral decision to the provision of services, child welfare decision-making research has primarily focused on the provision of ongoing child welfare services [16,24,28,34] and the decision to place children out-of-home [24,35–37]. The applicability and generalizability of the available extant service referral research to the Ontario child welfare context is limited by the lack of uniformity in several aspects of studies, including methodology, sample, variable type, definition of referral to services, the types of services referred to, the country of origin, and the broader policy and practice contexts. For example, Villigrana examined the factors that influence a referral to mental health services for child welfare-involved children by both court social workers and child welfare social workers in California by using case abstraction of closed court cases [38]. There were no significant predictors found for the decision to refer children to mental health services by child welfare social workers; however, significant predictors for mental health service referrals for court social workers have included the child remaining in their home and multiple types of abuse. Factors associated with service referrals have been found to differ by ethnicity [5]. For instance, a substantiation decision was more likely to result in a service referral for white families than for black families [5]. When compared to African American families, Hispanic families have been found to be more likely to be referred to psychosocial services than services that relate to basic needs, such as housing [10]. Amongst children with a developmental disability, a report of emotional maltreatment and out-of-home placement were two factors that increased the likelihood of a service referral for a formal assessment [39]. The likelihood of a referral to developmental services was more likely for cases in which the child welfare system had determined a need for services and where children experienced sexual abuse [40].There is a dearth of research that explores service referrals for infants and young children.

1.4. International Comparisons and Context

The majority of research exploring service referrals and/or utilization for child welfare-involved families originates from the United States, which has disparate policy, legislative, and practice contexts than Ontario, Canada. For instance, there are differences between the U.S. and Canada in how the knowledge of early childhood development has informed child welfare legislation and policies. In the U.S., amendments were made in 2003 to the Child Abuse and Prevention Act (CAPTA) in recognition of the importance of early intervention for young child welfare-involved children [11,40]. Funded under Part C of the Individuals with Disabilities Education Improvement Act (IDEA), states were required to develop referral procedures to early intervention services for children aged 0 to 3 years who were involved in a substantiated case of child maltreatment [11,40]. In 2011, the Child and Family Services Improvement and Innovations Act was introduced and this legislation required state reporting of activities involving young children in the child welfare system [41]. Moreover, in contrast to the U.S., child welfare in Canada is not governed by federal legislation, but legislation that is specific to each province and territory [42,43]. Ontario's child welfare legislative mandate gives central and equal consideration to the notions of both protection and well-being [44]; however, there are no policies that address early intervention for infants and young children who come into contact with the child welfare system, nor is there mandated referral legislation. Although there is an existing policy orientation in support of differential response models, wide-scale programs have yet to be implemented in Ontario [16,45]. In contrast, several states in the U.S. have undergone Differential Response reforms, which emphasize family assessment, parental involvement, and needs-driven service [46]. In comparison to families that undergo investigations, families that are offered services through an assessment approach have been found to be provided with a greater array of services [46].

Child welfare service models in Canada are not yet aligned with emerging investigative trends that suggest greater focus on the long-term impact of family dysfunction than immediate safety concerns [44].

Findings from the research on Canadian incidence studies at both the provincial and national levels suggest that infants are a unique subgroup of children involved with the child welfare system [16,28,34,37]. The age of children influences the risk of maltreatment and how the child welfare system subsequently responds to it [23,25,47]. Investigations involving infants are most likely to result in intensive service responses, including greater likelihood of receiving ongoing child welfare services and out-of-home placements [37]. Key drivers of service provision decisions differ by age. Caregiver risk factors have been found to drive the decision to provide ongoing child welfare services [16,28,34] and out-of-home placements for infants [48]. In contrast, child functioning concerns are key contributors for both decisions involving older children and adolescents [36,37]. These findings underscore the importance of exploring the unique mix of child, family, and broader environmental risks, protective factors, and needs that may emerge around specific ages and developmental stages [47]. The composition of services required to support families with infants should differ from those required to support families with older children [47]. Palusci found that infants and young children (0–5 years of age) involved with the child welfare system experienced different risk factors and services than those of older children [49]. There is a dearth of research exploring types of services offered to families who have had involvement with the child welfare system [10].

1.5. Research Questions

The state of the literature suggests that the child welfare decision to refer families to services warrants more focused attention, particularly given the salience of this decision to infants and their families within a Canadian child welfare context. There is no study that has specifically examined the service referral decision for infants and families who have been investigated by the child welfare system; nor, has there been an age-specific exploration of the patterns and types of services families have been referred to in a Canadian context. An understanding of the clinical profile infants and their families, their needs, and the child welfare system's response is critical to developing targeted, appropriate, and effective interventions. As a result of the significant gaps in the knowledge base, this exploratory study uses the Ontario Incidence Study of Reported Child Abuse and Neglect-2013 (OIS-2013) [50] to answer the following questions:

1. What are the characteristics (child, caregiver, household, case, and short-term service outcomes) of maltreatment-related investigations of children that are infants (less than 1) and do these characteristics differ when compared to other age groups, including, preschool aged (1–3), early school-aged (4–7), pre-adolescent (8–11), and adolescent (12–15) children investigated by the child welfare system across Ontario?
2. Which characteristics are associated with the decision to refer infants and families for supportive services following maltreatment-related investigations?
3. What are the types of supportive services that families of infants and older children are referred to?

The OIS is currently the only source of provincially aggregated child welfare data in Ontario. The OIS is also the only source of data that includes whether a child welfare worker made a referral for supportive services during the investigative period. The central objective of this study is to better understand the unique characteristics of infants and their families by exploring differences between infants and other age groups, and to build on the evolving research on factors related to service provision with this particularly vulnerable subpopulation of children. Understanding factors associated with child welfare service referral decisions for infants, and age-specific trends for the broader population of children, is important to strategically addressing and targeting child and family needs. This research provides a snapshot of the risk factors, child and family needs, and the supportive services that families are referred to at the conclusion of an initial child welfare investigation. Given the dearth of research on infants and the decision to provide service referrals within a Canadian child welfare context, this exploratory analysis is warranted and an important step for future research.

2. Materials and Methods

2.1. Sample

A secondary analysis of the 2013 cycle of the Ontario Incidence Study of Reported Child Abuse and Neglect (OIS) was conducted. The OIS-2013 is the fifth provincial study to examine provincial estimates of the incidence of reported child maltreatment and characteristics of the children and families investigated by the child protection system in Ontario. The OIS is a serial survey conducted with child welfare workers regarding their investigations of child maltreatment. The study is cross-sectional. The OIS utilizes a three-stage sampling design to select a representative sample of 17 child welfare agencies from a provincial list of 46 child welfare agencies [51]. Cases opened between 1 October 2013 and 31 December 2013 of the study cycle were eligible for inclusion in the study. Children not reported to child welfare services, screened out reports, and new allegations on open cases at the time of selection were not included in the OIS-2013. The three-month study period is considered optimal for participation and compliance with study procedures [51].

Maltreatment-related investigations included in the OIS-2013 are comprised of two types: (1) where there is no specific concern about past maltreatment but future risk of maltreatment is being assessed (risk-only); and (2) where maltreatment may have occurred. Maltreatment-related investigations, regardless of their substantiation status were included in this analysis. Children over 15 years of age, siblings not investigated, and children who were investigated for non-maltreatment concerns were excluded from the sample.

Child welfare cases in Ontario are counted as families. There were 3118 cases opened at the family-level during the 3-month period. The final stage of the sampling consisted of identifying investigated children as a result of maltreatment concerns. There were a total of 5265 children investigated as a result of the identification of maltreatment concerns. Of those 5265 children investigated, 345 were infants. The University of Toronto provided ethics approval (protocol number 28580).

2.2. Study Weights

Provincial estimates were derived by applying full weights, which includes both annualization and regionalization weights. These procedures yielded a final weighted sample of 125,281 children investigated because of maltreatment-related concerns. This study focused specifically on maltreatment-related investigations involving infants (under the age of 1 year) and explored factors associated with the decision to provide a referral for supportive services at the conclusion of the investigation. The final provincial estimate was 7915 investigations involving infants. For a detailed description of the OIS-2013 methodology and weighting procedures, please see Fallon and colleagues [51].

2.3. Data Collection Instrument

Data for the OIS-2013 is collected directly from investigating child welfare workers using a three-page standardized data collection instrument, the Maltreatment Assessment Form. This form is completed at the conclusion of the initial investigation. The OIS-2013 had an item completion rate of over 99% for all items. The instrument collected clinical information that child welfare workers routinely gather as part of their initial investigation, such as: caregiver, infant, case characteristics, and short-term service dispositions, including whether a referral for supportive services had been made, and the types of services referred to. Child welfare workers were asked to indicate whether any referrals for services had been made for any family member at the end of the investigation. If so, workers were asked to indicate all referrals that applied. These referrals include internal referrals to a special program provided by the child welfare organization or to other agencies or services external to the child welfare organization.

2.4. Variable Selection

The decision to refer to services is a dichotomous variable. The variable definitions and codes used in this analysis are provided in Table 1. Clinical variables were chosen on their availability in the dataset and on the literature addressing factors related to the occurrence of child maltreatment and the child welfare system's response to infants.

Table 1. Variable definitions and codes.

Variable	Description	Measurement
Outcome		
Referral to supportive services	Workers were asked to indicate if a referral was made to any services internal to the child welfare system or externally to community services (e.g., parent support group) for any family member.	Dichotomous variable: 1 Referral for services 0 No referral for services
Predictors		
Child Characteristics		
Child sex	Worker identified the sex of the investigated child.	Dichotomous variable: 1 Male 0 Female
Child ethno-racial group	Workers were asked to indicate the ethno-racial background of the child (Black, Latin American, Arab, Aboriginal, Asian). Ethno-racial categories developed by Statistics Canada.	Dichotomous variable: 1 Ethnic minority 0 White
Child functioning	Workers were asked to note up to eighteen child functioning concerns. Six of eighteen dichotomous child functioning variables are relevant to infants: failure to meet developmental milestones, attachment issues, intellectual/developmental disability, FAS/FAE, positive toxicology at birth, physical disability. This analysis noted whether the worker examined at least one of these six concerns.	1 At least one child functioning concern noted. 0 No child functioning concerns noted
Caregiver Characteristics		
Primary caregiver age	Workers were asked to indicate the age category of the primary caregiver.	Categorical variable: 1 21 years and under 2 22 years and up
Primary caregiver risk factors	Workers could note up to nine functioning concerns for the primary caregiver. Concerns were: alcohol abuse, drug/solvent abuse, cognitive impairment, mental health issues, physical health issues, few social supports, victim of domestic violence, perpetrator of domestic violence, and history of foster care/group home.	Nine dichotomous variables: 1 Suspected or confirmed 0 No or unknown
Primary income of caregiver	Workers were asked to indicate the primary source of the primary caregiver's income.	Categorical variable: 1 Full time/Part time 0 Other benefits/unemployment/ No income
Household characteristics		
No second caregiver in the home	Workers were asked to describe up to two caregivers in the home. If there was only one caregiver described there was no second caregiver in the home.	Dichotomous variable: 1 No second caregiver in home 0 Second caregiver in home
Household hazards	Workers were asked to note if the following hazards were present in the home at the time of the investigation: accessible weapons, accessible drugs, production/trafficking of drugs, chemicals/solvents, used in drug production, other home injury hazards, and other home health hazards.	Dichotomous variable: 1 At least one household hazard 0 No household hazard
Household regularly runs out of money	Workers were asked to note if the household regularly runs out of money for food, housing and/or utilities in the last six months.	Dichotomous variable: 1 Noted 0 Not noted
Number of moves	Workers were asked to note the number of moves the household had in the past six months.	2 2 or more moves 1 One or more moves 0 None
Case characteristics		
Previous openings	Worker indicated if there were one or more previous child protection openings.	1 One or more previous openings. 0 No openings
Type of investigation	Workers were asked to indicate if the investigation was conducted for a specific maltreatment incident (maltreatment investigation), or if it was to assess a risk of maltreatment only (risk-only investigation).	1 Maltreatment investigation 2 Risk-only investigation

2.5. Analyitic Approach

Descriptive and bivariate analyses were conducted in order to explore and compare the profile of investigations involving infants (under the age of 1) to children in older age groups, including preschool (1–3), and early school-age (4–7), pre-adolescent (8–11), and adolescent (12–15) children in Ontario in 2013. Provincial incidence estimates were calculated by dividing the weighted estimates by the child population based upon 2011 Census data from Statistics Canada. Chi-square tests of significance were conducted using the normalized sample weight, which adjusts for the inflation of the chi-square statistic by the size of the estimate by weighing the estimate down to the original sample size. As Table 2 shows, infants were compared to four other age groups and the p-value was subsequently adjusted as a result (0.05/4 comparisons = 0.013). Thus, all significance tests for chi-square analyses conducted and shown in Table 2 were evaluated using the adjusted p-value ($p < 0.013$), resulting from the Bonferroni correction given the four multiple comparisons.

Multivariate analysis was conducted in order to explore which variables were significant with the decision to provide a service referral at the conclusion of maltreatment-related investigations involving infants. Prior to the logistic regression, bivariate chi-square analyses were conducted to explore associations between clinical and case characteristics and service referrals. Only variables that were significant at the bivariate level ($p < 0.05$) were included in the logistic regression model. Logistic regression was deemed an appropriate analysis strategy as the outcome variable is dichotomous and it can estimate the relationship between predictor variables with the likelihood or probability of an event occurring [52]. The cutoff point for the decision to refer to services was 0.57, which reflects the proportion of investigations referred for services for the infant population. This analysis did not include missing data in the bivariate or multivariate analysis. Unweighted data were used in the multivariate model to ensure unbiased results due to the inflation of significance due to a large sample size. All analyses were conducted using SPSS, version 23 (SPSS Inc., Chicago, IL, USA).

3. Results

Numerous distinctions emerged in child, primary caregiver, household, maltreatment, case characteristics, and service outcomes between infants and older children investigated in Ontario in 2013 (Figure 1, Table 2). In comparison to all other age groups, maltreatment-related investigations involving infants had the highest incidence of a service referral at 33.50 per 1000; followed by early school-aged children at 24.69 per 1000; preadolescents at 23.07 per 1000 investigations; pre-schoolers at 22.93 per 1000; and adolescents at 20.66 per 1000 (Figure 1). Incidence rates suggest that investigations involving adolescents were the least likely to result in the decision to provide a service referral for any family member, with a rate of 20.66 per 1000.

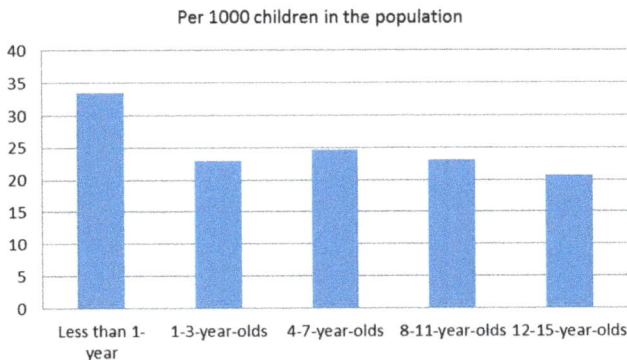

Figure 1. Incidence of a service referral for maltreatment-related investigations by child age.

Table 2. Prevalence and bivariate analyses of investigation characteristics by child age for maltreatment-related investigations in Ontario in 2013.

Variable	Child Age					χ^2
	Less than 1Year- Old $n = 7915$	1–3- Year- Olds $n = 21,801$	4–7- Year- Olds $n = 36,730$	8–11- Year- Olds $n = 29,907$	12–15- Year- Olds $n = 28,928$	
Child characteristics						
Child Sex (female)	49.30%	49.40%	48.50%	45.10%	51.30%	NS
Child Ethnicity						
Ethnic minority	30.90%	36.10%	35.60%	35.30%	34.90%	NS
White	69.10%	63.90%	64.40%	64.70%	65.10%	
Child Functioning Concerns						
At Least One Child Functioning Concern	7.80%	10.10%	17.10%	21.30%	26.20%	$p < 0.001$ b;c;d
Primary caregiver characteristics						
Primary Caregiver Age						
21 years or under	31.30%	9.80%	0.70%	0%	0.10%	$p < 0.001$ a;b;c;d
22 years or more	68.70%	90.20%	99.30%	100%	99.90%	
Primary Caregiver Risk Factors						
Alcohol Abuse	10.60%	6.50%	6.80%	7.30%	5.70%	$p < 0.01$ d
Drug/Solvent Use	18.80%	8.60%	6.20%	6.40%	4.10%	$p < 0.001$ a;b;c;d
Cognitive Impairment	8.80%	3.90%	3.80%	4.30%	2.60%	$p < 0.01$ a;c $p < 0.001$ b;d
Mental Health Issues	31.10%	22.10%	19.00%	19.50%	20.60%	$p < 0.01$ a; $p < 0.001$ b;c;d
Physical Health Issues	5.90%	4.70%	5.60%	6.80%	9.00%	NS
Few Social Supports	32.80%	30.90%	22.30%	21.50%	24.50%	$p < 0.001$ b;c $p < 0.01$ d
Victim of IPV	37.60%	33.50%	25.60%	24.80%	20.00%	$p < 0.001$ b;c;d
Perpetrator of IPV	10.80%	11.80%	7.30%	7.80%	6.10%	$p < 0.01$ d
History of Foster Care	13.00%	7.40%	4.10%	4.00%	2.20%	$p < 0.01$ a $p < 0.001$ b;c;d
At least one caregiver functioning concern	74.30%	63.10%	52.30%	52.80%	52.30%	$p < 0.001$ a;b;c;d
Household characteristics						
No Second Caregiver in Home	30.40%	31.20%	37.40%	32.60%	38.10%	$p < 0.01$d
Primary Income						
Full-time/part-time/seasonal	12.80%	35.70%	49.60%	57.20%	64.00%	$p < 0.001$ a;b;c;d
Other Benefits/Unemployment/ No income	87.20%	64.30%	50.40%	42.80%	36.00%	
At Least One Household Hazard	8.80%	4.80%	4.10%	5.10%	3.40%	$p < 0.01$ a;b $p < 0.001$ d
Household Regularly Runs Out of Money	15.70%	9.20%	7.40%	7.90%	7.30%	$p < 0.01$ a $p < 0.001$ b;c;d
Number of Moves						
No Moves	50.00%	62.20%	69.80%	77.00%	79.10%	$p < 0.001$ a $p < 0.001$ b;c;d
One Move	32.50%	29.80%	25.00%	19.00%	17.10%	
Two or More Moves	17.40%	8.00%	5.20%	4.00%	3.80%	
Maltreatment characteristics						
Type of Maltreatment-Related Investigation						$p < 0.001$ a;b;c;d
Maltreatment						
Physical Abuse	2.10%	12.40%	24.00%	24.30%	21.00%	
Sexual Abuse	1.20%	1.10%	3.80%	3.60%	5.02%	
Neglect	20.40%	20.50%	21.60%	21.60%	21.70%	
Emotional Maltreatment	5.40%	7.40%	8.30%	8.20%	10.60%	
Exposure to (IPV)	31.20%	31.30%	24.40%	23.90%	20.40%	
Risk	39.80%	27.30%	18.00%	18.30%	21.20%	
Case characteristics and service outcomes						
At least one previous case opening (family level)	43.60%	60.50%	63.20%	68.20%	72.70%	$p < 0.001$ a;b;c;d
Child previously investigated for alleged maltreatment (child level)	16.90%	45.90%	56.90%	64.20%	67.70%	$p < 0.001$ a;b;c;d
Opened for ongoing services	39.80%	25.70%	21.60%	23.60%	26.30%	$p < 0.001$ a;b;c;d
Child welfare court	8.80%	1.90%	1.90%	1.50%	3.30%	$p < 0.001$ a;b;c;d
Placement	8.60%	1.20%	2.20%	2.80%	5.90%	$p < 0.001$ a;b;c
Investigations with a service referral	57.2%	46.0%	39.0%	45.4%	46.3%	$p < 0.001$ a;b;c;d

Source: 2013 Ontario Incidence Study of Reported Child Abuse and Neglect; a = statistically significant difference in service referrals between infants (less than 1 year old) and 1–3-year-olds. b = statistically significant difference in service referrals between infants and 4–7-year-olds. c = statistically significant difference in service referrals between infants and 8–11-year-olds. d = statistically significant difference in service referrals between infants and 12–15-year-olds ($p < 0.01$; $p < 0.001$), NS = not statistically significant. Chi-square analyses were conducted with the normalized sample weight. Estimated number of provincial investigations, $n = 125,281$.

3.1. Child Characteristics

Descriptive and chi-square analyses revealed many differences between infants and the other four age groups (Table 2). The distribution of child characteristics, including sex and ethnicity are similar across the five different age groups (Table 2). The likelihood of a child welfare worker identifying a child functioning concern increased with age (Table 2 and Figure 2). Infants were significantly less likely to have a child functioning concern identified when compared to children who were early school-aged (4–7), pre-adolescent (8–11), and adolescent (12–15). Infants had the lowest incidence at a rate of 4.53 per 1000. In contrast, adolescents (12–15) had the highest incidence rate at 11.93 per 1000.

Per 1000 children in the population

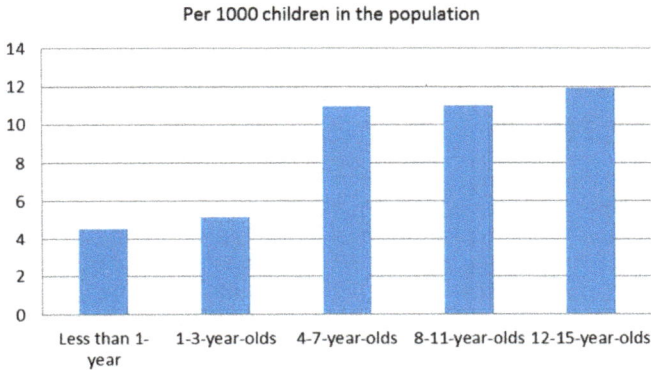

Figure 2. Incidence of a child functioning concern in maltreatment-related investigations.

3.2. Primary Caregiver Characteristics and Risk Factors

Infants had the highest incidence of caregivers identified as having at least one risk factor, with a rate of 43.44 per 1000 (Figure 3). Early school-aged children followed next with an incidence rate of 33.64 per 1000, preschoolers have an incidence rate of 32.33 per 1000, and preadolescents have an incident rate of 27.17 per 1000. Adolescents have the lowest incidence rate of caregivers identified with at least one caregiver risk factor at a rate of 23.78 per 1000.

Per 1000 children in the population

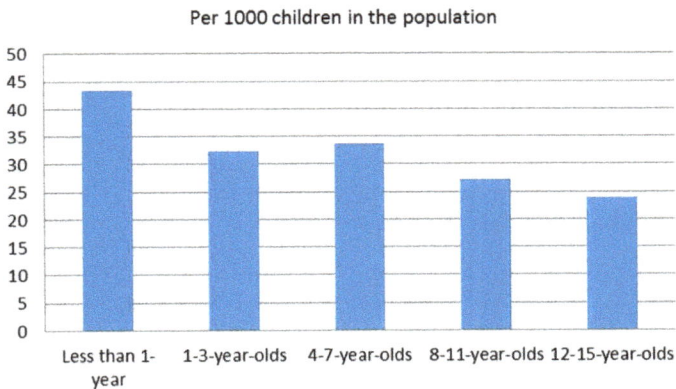

Figure 3. Incidence of a caregiver risk factor in maltreatment-related investigations in Ontario 2013.

Chi square tests (Table 2) revealed caregivers of infants were significantly more likely to be younger (21 years of age or under) than caregivers of children in each of the four older age groups. Caregivers of infants were also significantly more likely to be identified as having the following risk factors: drug solvent use, cognitive impairment, mental health issues, having a history of foster care, and having at least one caregiver risk factor identified. The three most common caregiver risk factors identified for caregivers of infants were being a victim of IPV, few social supports, and having a mental health issue (Table 2).

3.3. Household Characteristics

Infants were most frequently identified as living in households with at least one hazard, regularly running out of money, and moving two or more times. Chi-square analyses also indicated that infants were significantly more likely to be identified to be living in a household that regularly ran out of money for basic necessities than families of older children.

3.4. Maltreatment, Case Characteristics, and Short-Term Service Outcomes

When compared to all other age groups, infants were most likely to be involved in investigations where there was no specific incident of maltreatment alleged, but there was an allegation of future risk of maltreatment. Infants and pre-school aged children were most frequently investigated for exposure to IPV. Neglect was the most common type of investigated maltreatment, with minimal variation across age groups. Moreover, in comparison to each of the four older age groups, investigations involving infants were significantly more likely to result in court involvement and a transfer to ongoing child welfare services. With the exception of adolescents, investigations involving infants were significantly more likely to result in an out-of-home placement for all other age groups. Infants and adolescents were among the age groups with the highest prevalence of out-of-home placement post-investigation.

3.5. Characteristics Related with Service Referrals for Maltreatment-Related Investigations Involving Infants

Chi-square analyses were conducted in order to determine which child, caregiver, household, and case characteristics influenced the decision to provide a referral for maltreatment-related investigations involving infants. Table 3 shows the characteristics of maltreatment-related investigations involving infants and the eight variables that were significantly associated with the decision to provide referrals for supportive services: the identification of a child functioning issue, younger primary caregiver age, drug/solvent use; few social supports, at least one household hazard, regularly running out of money; and, greater number of moves. The eight variables found to be significant in relation to service referrals were then placed in the binary logistic regression model.

Table 3. Referral-related characteristics in maltreatment-related investigations involving infants referred for services in Ontario in 2013.

Variable	Referral for Services		
	Estimate	%	χ^2
Child Characteristics			
Child sex			
Male	2302	57.6%	0.01
Female	2228	57.3%	
Child ethnicity			
Ethnic minority	1212	50.6%	3.65
White	3310	61.8%	
Child functioning issue			
At least one identified	472	76.9%	4.41 *

Table 3. *Cont.*

Variable	Referral for Services		
Caregiver Characteristics			
Primary caregiver age			
21 years and under	1638	66.4%	5.29 *
22 years and up	2855	52.8%	
Primary caregiver risk factors			
Alcohol Abuse	556	66.0%	1.15
Drug/Solvent Use	1087	73.0%	7.79 **
Cognitive Impairment	488	69.8%	2.16
Mental Health Issues	1590	64.7%	3.23
Physical Health Issues	321	68.9%	1.03
Few Social Supports	1743	67.1%	6.29 *
Victim of IPV	2124	71.3%	15.99 ***
Perpetrator of IPV	517	60.6%	0.23
History of Foster Care	580	56.3%	0.04
Primary income of caregiver			
Full time/Part time	457	48.3%	3.12
Other benefits/unemployment/no income	4016	62.2%	
Household characteristics			
No second caregiver in the home	1470	61.1%	0.96
Household hazards	566	85.1%	9.18 ***
Household regularly runs out of money	749	72.7%	3.86 *
Number of moves			
None	1499	46.0%	24.45 ***
One move	1604	75.6%	
Two or more moves	849	74.6%	
Case characteristics			
Previous openings	2096	60.8%	1.26
Type of investigation			
Maltreatment	2598	54.5%	1.53
Risk	1932	61.3%	

Source: 2013 Ontario Incidence Study of Reported Child Abuse and Neglect; * $p < 0.05$; ** $p < 0.01$; *** $p < 0.001$.

3.6. Predictors of Service Referral for Maltreatment-Related Investigations Involving Infants: Logistic Regression Analysis

There were two primary caregiver characteristics that contributed to the prediction of a service referral for infants in the final model: being a victim of IPV and primary caregiver age. Thus, infants' exposure to IPV and having a younger caregiver increased the likelihood of a service referral (Table 4). Having a caregiver who was a victim of IPV was the largest contributor to the decision to refer to specialized services. Having a primary caregiver aged 21 years or younger, in comparison to having a primary caregiver 22 years or older, more than doubled the odds of being referred for services (OR = 2.54, $p < 0.01$). The presence of IPV among primary caregivers increased the likelihood of a service referral being made by a factor of 2.81 (OR = 2.81, $p < 0.01$). The omnibus tests of model coefficients χ^2 (8) = 39.24, $p < 0.001$ indicates that the model was significant. The model accounted for approximately 20.0% of the variance on the outcome (Nagelkerke R^2 = 0.20).

Table 4. Logistic regression model predicting service referrals for maltreatment-related investigations involving infants in Ontario in 2013.

Variable	B (SE)	Wald	OR	95% CI
Child characteristics				
At least one child functioning issue	0.39 (0.53)	0.53	1.47	0.52–4.16
Primary caregiver characteristics				
Primary Caregiver Age (22 years or more)				
21 years or under	0.93 (0.32)	8.52	2.54 **	1.36–4.75
Primary Caregiver Risk Factors				
Drug/Solvent Abuse	0.32 (0.40)	0.65	1.38	0.63–3.02
Few Social Supports	0.57 (0.32)	3.16	1.76	0.94–3.28
Victim of IPV	1.04 (0.31)	11.32	2.83 **	1.54–5.18
Household characteristics				
At Least One Household Hazard	0.73 (0.59)	1.54	2.07	0.66–6.51
Household Regularly Runs Out of Money	0.12 (0.41)	0.08	1.12	0.52–2.42
Number of Moves (No Moves)				
One Move	0.45 (0.32)	2.04	1.60	0.85–2.91
Two or More Moves	0.06 (0.50)	0.16	1.06	0.42–2.67
Omnibus Chi-Square Test	39.24			
p-value	$p < 0.001$			
Nagelkerke R-square	0.20			
% Classified correctly	67.6			
−2 Log Likelihood	301.54			

Source: 2013 Ontario Incidence Study of Reported Child Abuse and Neglect; SE, Standard error; OR, Odds Ratio; CI, Confidence Interval; * $p < 0.05$; ** $p < 0.01$; *** $p < 0.001$.

3.7. Referral to Supportive Services

General areas for possible referrals to supportive services included: parenting and family support; addiction and mental health support; physical health; IPV, legal and victim support; income, food and housing support; cultural services; speech and language; and, recreational services. As Table 5 shows, interesting patterns emerged in the types of referrals provided by child welfare workers by age group. In comparison to all other age groups, families of infants were most commonly referred to a parent support group and in-home family or parenting counseling, and/or addiction counseling. Amongst families of infants, parenting and family support was the most common type of service referred to by child welfare workers.

Table 5. Type of service referrals in maltreatment-related investigations by age group in Ontario in 2013.

Variable	Child Age				
Type of Service(s) Referred to	Less than 1- Year Old *n* = 4530	1–3- Year-Olds *n* = 9755	4–7- Year-Olds *n* = 14,104	8–11- Year-Olds *n* = 13,400	12–15- Year-Olds *n* = 13,148
Parenting or family support					
Parent support group	22.7%	14.2%	16.1%	10.9%	14.9%
In-home family/parent counseling	20.8%	12.8%	13.5%	11.9%	11.9%
Other family/parent counseling	22.6%	35.8%	43.4%	44.8%	53.8%
Child or day care	6.3%	16.0%	5.8%	1.7%	0.8%
Addiction and mental health support					
Drug or alcohol counseling	17.4%	14.3%	11.3%	11.9%	11.2%
Psychiatric or psychological services	10.4%	14.5%	15.4%	16.0%	19.5%
Physical health support (medical/dental)	6.4%	6.7%	4.4%	5.3%	5.0%
IPV, legal and victim support					
IPV services	24.0%	24.7%	19.6%	18.1%	14.0%
Victim support program	4.7%	11.1%	9.4%	7.3%	6.4%
Legal	13.3%	16.5%	9.8%	10.2%	7.1%

Table 5. *Cont.*

Variable	Child Age				
Type of Service(s) Referred to	Less than 1- Year Old *n* = 4530	1–3- Year- Olds *n* = 9755	4–7- Year- Olds *n* = 14,104	8–11- Year- Olds *n* = 13,400	12–15- Year- Olds *n* = 13,148
Income, food and housing support					
Welfare or social assistance	7.8%	6.0%	3.1%	1.4%	3.3%
Food bank	7.8%	7.0%	6.4%	5.7%	6.0%
Shelter services	5.5%	11.4%	7.0%	4.2%	5.7%
Housing	9.6%	12.8%	4.8%	6.5%	4.0%
Cultural services	2.7%	2.8%	3.4%	4.1%	5.7%
Speech or language	0.8%	5.6%	1.9%	1.2%	1.1%
Recreational services	3.7%	6.7%	5.3%	5.9%	4.2%

Source: Ontario Incidence Study of Reported Child Abuse and Neglect 2013; Percentages do not add up to 100% because investigating child welfare workers could identify more than one service referred to.

Families with infants were most likely to receive a referral for drug or alcohol counseling; whereas families with adolescents were most likely to receive referrals for mental health. Overall, families of infants and preschool aged children were most likely to receive referrals for supports for meeting their basic needs, and included income, food, and housing supports. When compared to families of children in older age groups, families with younger children (i.e., infants and preschool aged children) were almost equally likely to be referred for IPV supports.

4. Discussion

Utilizing a Canadian provincial dataset, this study corroborates and extends the existing research. The findings highlight the distinct profile of infants and families investigated by the child welfare system. When comparing maltreatment-related investigations of infants to older children, numerous differences emerged with respect to risks, service needs, the child welfare system's response, and the types of supportive services referred to by the child welfare system. The findings of this study also provide a broad understanding of the clinical factors that drive the decision to provide a referral to services for infants and their families. The majority of investigations involving infants received a service referral. When compared to older children, maltreatment-related investigations involving infants were significantly more likely to result in a referral for supportive services. These findings are indicative of the child welfare system's recognition of the complex challenges families of infants are contending with and the importance and necessity of working with services in the community to address them. When comparing caregivers of infants to those of older children, caregivers of infants were significantly more likely to be identified as having at least one functioning issue. Maltreatment-related investigations involving infants were significantly more likely to have an investigating worker identify primary caregiver risk factors that include drug/solvent use, cognitive impairment, and a history of foster care. Alcohol abuse, drug/solvent use, cognitive impairments, mental health issues, few social supports, being a victim of IPV, and having a history of foster care were risk factors that were more common for caregivers of infants.

When compared to older children, infants were more likely to live in homes that regularly ran out of money for basic necessities, such as food, shelter, and utilities. These findings are consistent with research indicating that families with younger children tend to experience greater socio-economic hardships than older children [36,37]. This finding is concerning given that the literature suggests that low socio-economic status is linked to poor developmental outcomes for younger children as a result of its detrimental impact on the quality of the infant-caregiver relationship [53]. Poverty has also been identified as a risk factor for neglect [29]. This study found that neglect was the primary form of maltreatment alleged in approximately 1 in every 5 maltreatment-related investigations for each age group. The rapidity of brain development during infancy makes infants particularly susceptible to the profound and widespread developmental effects of neglect [29].

Infants were also significantly more likely to be investigated for reasons other than specific incidents of alleged maltreatment. Although the type of investigation (risk-only versus maltreatment) was not associated with the decision to provide a referral in this study, previous research suggests that risk-only investigations present with similar household and poverty-related concerns as maltreatment investigations [54]. This raises issues with respect to the operationalization of child welfare's dual mandate of child safety and well-being for infants, particularly within the context of traditional service delivery models that emphasize protection. A child safety focus tends to prioritize the assessment of risk; whereas, a focus on well-being prioritizes the assessment of child and family needs [50]. Child welfare service decisions, including the decision to refer to services, should be based on a comprehensive assessment that includes consideration of both risk and needs [50]. This study corroborates previous research that suggests that infants and their families are the recipients of the child welfare system's most intensive responses [37]. When compared to older children, infants were significantly more likely to be transferred to ongoing services and to be the subject of a court application. Both infants had the highest proportion of out-of-home placements, followed by adolescents. Previous research has found that infants are more likely than older children to be placed out-of-home [37]; however, it is important to note that the vast majority of infants in this study (over 90%) remained in the home following a maltreatment-related investigation. Commonly, infants who remain at home following alleged maltreatment experience high rates of re-reporting [55]. Research examining the re-reporting of infants and children following maltreatment-related investigations that considers the Ontario child welfare context is important to informing prevention and intervention efforts [56].

Two factors were significant in predicting the decision to refer to services and both were associated with the primary caregiver: being a victim of IPV and younger caregiver age. As in Jud, Fallon, and Trocmé's study, the presence of IPV had a significant impact on the decision to refer to services [24]. Having a caregiver who was a victim of IPV was the most common caregiver risk factor identified by investigating child welfare workers for all age groups, with the exception of adolescents. In keeping with the findings of Fallon and colleagues, IPV exposure in this study was found to be the most commonly identified concern in maltreatment-related investigations involving infants in Ontario [16]. The finding that service referral decisions were also significantly associated with younger caregiver age is consistent with previous Canadian research [24] and the broader literature indicating that young caregiver age is a risk factor for maltreatment and is associated with the decision to provide ongoing services [16,28,34,57]. It is notable that many variables (e.g., child functioning concern, primary caregiver drug/solvent use, primary caregiver with few social supports) did not contribute to the decision to provide a service referral for infants. It appears that child welfare workers were most clinically concerned about the impact of IPV and younger caregiver age on caregiving skills and ability to meet infants' needs. Previous research from Ontario conducted by Fallon and colleagues suggests that a differential systems response is required for IPV and this should depend on the type of exposure and the constellation of other risk factors at the child, family, and household levels [58]. Further research is required to better understand the child welfare response to IPV in a Canadian context [58].

The absence of association between caregiver mental health and service referral at the bivariate level is not in keeping with broader Canadian research on infants that has linked caregiver mental health to other service provision decisions, such as the decision to provide ongoing services [16,34], and the decision to place infants out-of-home [48]. Moreover, there is a well-established body of research that suggests that caregiver functioning issues, such as chronic depression, may act to compromise the quality of the infant-caregiver relationship and negatively impact short-term and long-term development [59]. Socio-economic hardship risk variables (e.g., running out of money for basic necessities, primary income, unsafe housing/household hazards) did not seemingly impact the likelihood of service referrals in this model. It may be that the measures informing socio-economic disadvantage are somewhat crude and socio-economic status is generally quite low for many families that come to the attention of the child welfare system in Ontario.

Disparities in the decision to provide and utilize services have been linked to child race and ethnicity [5,10,60]. In this study, child ethnicity was not significant at the bivariate level. This is in keeping with Jud, Fallon, and Trocmé's study that found that ethnicity did not influence the decision to provide ongoing services or a referral for supportive services [24]. The role of child race in service referral decision-making is not well understood [5] Further research is needed to explore racial and ethnic disparities in service provision decisions, including the decision to refer to services regarding infants within a Canadian child welfare context.

In keeping with previous research [16], this study revealed that when compared to older children, infants in Ontario are less likely to be identified as having a child functioning issue. Although found to be significantly associated with service referrals at the bivariate level for infants, the identification of a child functioning concern did not predict a service referral in the multivariate model. The literature compellingly suggests that the mental health needs of infants and young children involved with the child welfare system are under-identified and untreated. Referral to appropriate services for families and children starts with the accurate identification of needs. There is no comprehensive or systematic developmental screening strategy in place in Ontario for infants involved with the child welfare system. Standardized, reliable, and valid measures may assist child welfare workers in the assessment and identification of need of early intervention services. There were age-specific differences in the types of services families were referred to by investigating child welfare workers. This study revealed that families of infants and young children (0–3 years old) were most commonly referred to services that relate to IPV and parenting/family support, such as support groups and/or counselling. Infants and younger children (ages 0–3 years) were also more commonly referred to income, food, and housing support services (e.g., social assistance, food bank, and shelter services) than older children. The importance of adopting a differential approach to child welfare policy, practice, and research that considers child age has been forwarded and is supported by the findings of this study [61]. Ontario has not yet implemented wide-scale programs with respect to differential response options [16,45]. Together with other studies, these findings lead to questioning whether an alternative or differential response approach with infants should be a consideration given their distinct clinical profile, risks, and need for supportive services.

In principle, service referrals should be primarily driven by case or clinical factors; however, child welfare service decisions are complex and can be influenced by factors at other levels, including worker, organizational, and the broader environment [62]. In addition, organization-level factors and regional variations have been found to influence the likelihood of service referrals [24]. The availability and accessibility of services may also be influencing child welfare workers' decisions to refer to services to and the types of services are referred to. As such, both availability and accessibility may be influenced by geographic location, which may in turn influence the ability of families to utilize community services [63]. Location may be a proxy measure for several underlying organizational constructs, including differential access to resources and partnerships between social service agencies and child welfare organizations [64]. Differences in child welfare services and geographic location or jurisdiction have not been adequately addressed in the literature [64]. Thus, influences at the organizational and structural levels require further research, particularly with respect to maltreatment-related investigations involving infants [24].

In Ontario, infant and childhood mental health has been identified as, " ... an issue that requires further policy development to ensure the availability and accessibility of optimal and consistent services across the province" (p. 5) [65]. To date, there is no provincial strategy that has focused on the mental health needs of infants and young children in Canada [65]. A key recommendation made for immediate policy development includes the provision of targeted supports to populations at-risk and working with an inter-generational intervention model [65]. Clinton and colleagues noted that infant-caregiver dyad is not the primary client focus in Ontario services, as infants and caregivers are treated as distinct entities [65].

Study Limitations

There are several limitations to this study that must be considered when interpreting the results. Data collected from the OIS is collected directly from the investigating child welfare worker and are not independently verified. The data is representative of an investigative period of thirty days after the case has opened. The study is cross-sectional and does not track longer-term service events that occurred beyond the initial investigation. The three-month sampling period is considered optimum to ensuring high participation rates and compliance with study procedures [51]. Consultations with service providers have indicated that case activity during the three-month period is reflective of the year; however, follow-up studies are needed to explore the extent of the possible impact of seasonal variation in types of cases reported on estimates [51]. The sample size of maltreatment-related investigations involving infants may have precluded some significant relationships from emerging. Types of services referred to were categorized broadly by family, not by child or caregiver, and provide a broad understanding of risk and needs. The OIS does not track specific referral actions or strategies used by child welfare workers (e.g., providing families with names and numbers, assisted caregiver with the referral). The OIS does not track whether services were received as a result of referral made by the worker during the investigative period. The OIS tracks whether a referral has been made and they type of services referred to. It is unknown whether families were engaged in other community services during this period. Moreover, the amount of variance explained by this model was small, with a large proportion of variance unaccounted for.

5. Conclusions

This study contributes to the minimal knowledge base relating to infants served by the child welfare system within a Canadian context. Despite the study limitations in tracking the progress of infants through the child welfare system, this study marks an important step to moving towards a better understanding of what investigations will effectively address the needs of vulnerable infants and their families. To date, the OIS is the only source of aggregated data in the province of Ontario and the findings are a reminder of the importance of provincial data in exploring and advocating for possible gaps in supports and resources for child-welfare involved children. Child welfare policy is set by the provincial government that also sets policies and funds for other allied sectors (e.g., children's mental health) that are integral to effective service provision. Greater understanding of the factors associated with service referrals and the types of services referred to can assist in aligning, organizing, and targeting child welfare and community services to address the risks and needs of child-welfare involved children and families.

A referral for services can be viewed as a critical step to enhancing infants' safety and well-being, and should be predicated upon the accurate identification of infant and family risks and needs. There are concerns that the child welfare system missing opportunities to identify, and thereby, ameliorate infants' well-being given the extant literature and this study's findings of low identification of infant functioning. Further research within a Canadian context is necessary in order to address these concerns. Moreover, adequately addressing infant well-being requires services that are accessible, available, and effective. As the findings suggest, infants are a distinctly vulnerable group of children involved with the child welfare system and require urgent and coherent attention at policy and practice levels within the field of child welfare and across multiple sectors.

Acknowledgments: We acknowledge the support of the Social Sciences and Humanities Research Council (#950-231186).

Author Contributions: B.F. is the Principal Investigator of the OIS-2013. J.F. synthesized the literature, conducted data analyses and interpretation, and wrote the manuscript. All authors contributed to data interpretation and had input into the manuscript.

Conflicts of Interest: There are no conflicts of interest.

Brain Sci. **2017**, *7*, 101

References

1. Simon, J.D.; Brooks, D. Identifying families with complex needs after an initial child abuse investigation: A comparison of demographics and needs related to domestic violence, mental health, and substance use. *Child Abuse Negl.* **2017**, *67*, 294–304. [CrossRef] [PubMed]
2. Simon, J.D.; Brooks, D. Post-investigation service need and utilization among families at risk of maltreatment. *Child. Youth Serv. Rev.* **2016**, *69*, 223–232. [CrossRef]
3. Stein, R.E.K.; Hurlburt, M.S.; Heneghan, A.M.; Zhang, J.; Kerker, B.; Landsverk, J.; Horwitz, S.M. For Better or Worse? Change in Service Use by Children Investigated by Child Welfare Over a Decade. *Acad. Pediatr.* **2016**, *16*, 240–246. [CrossRef] [PubMed]
4. Marsh, J.C.; Ryan, J.P.; Choi, S.; Testa, M.F. Integrated services for families with multiple problems: Obstacles to family reunification. *Child. Youth Serv. Rev.* **2006**, *28*, 1074–1087. [CrossRef]
5. Font, S.A. Service referral patterns among black and white families involved with child protective services. *J. Public Child Welf.* **2013**, *7*, 370–391. [CrossRef]
6. Choi, S.; Ryan, J.P. Co-occurring problems for substance abusing mothers in child welfare: Matching services to improve family reunification. *Child. Youth Serv. Rev.* **2007**, *29*, 1395–1410. [CrossRef]
7. Ryan, J.P.; Schuerman, J.R. Matching family problems with specific family preservation services: A study of service effectiveness. *Child. Youth Serv. Rev.* **2004**, *26*, 347–372. [CrossRef]
8. National Scientific Council on the Developing Child. *Establishing a Level Foundation for Life: Mental Health Begins in Early Childhood*; Harvard University, Center on the Developing Child: Cambridge, MA, USA, 2008.
9. Perry, B.D. Examining child maltreatment through a neurodevelopmental lens: Clinical applications of the neurosequential model of therapeutics. *J. Loss Trauma* **2009**, *14*, 240–255. [CrossRef]
10. Lovato-Hermann, K.; Dellor, E.; Tam, C.C.; Curry, S.; Freisthler, B. Racial disparities in service referrals for families in the child welfare system. *J. Public Child Welf.* **2017**, *11*, 133–149. [CrossRef]
11. McCrae, J.S.; Cahalane, H.; Fusco, R.A. Directions for developmental screening in child welfare based on the ages and stages questionnaires. *Child. Youth Serv. Rev.* **2011**, *33*, 1412–1418. [CrossRef]
12. Casanueva, C.E.; Cross, T.P.; Ringeisen, H. Developmental needs and individualized family service plans among infants and toddlers in the child welfare system. *Child Maltreat.* **2008**, *13*, 245–258. [CrossRef] [PubMed]
13. Burns, B.J.; Phillips, S.D.; Wagner, H.R.; Barth, R.P.; Kolko, D.J.; Campbell, Y.; Landsverk, J. Mental health need and access to mental health services by youths involved with child welfare: A national survey. *J. Am. Acad. Child Adolesc. Psychiatry* **2004**, *43*, 960–970. [CrossRef] [PubMed]
14. McCue Horwitz, S.; Hurlburt, M.S.; Heneghan, A.; Zhang, J.; Rolls-Reutz, J.; Fisher, E.; Landsverk, J.; Stein, R.E.K. Mental health problems in young children investigated by U.S. child welfare agencies. *J. Am. Acad. Child Adolesc. Psychiatry* **2012**, *51*, 572–581. [CrossRef] [PubMed]
15. Ringeisen, H.; Casanueva, C.; Cross, T.P.; Urato, M. Mental health and special education services at school entry for children who were involved with the child welfare system as infants. *J. Emot. Behav. Disord.* **2009**, *17*, 177–192. [CrossRef]
16. Fallon, B.; Ma, J.; Allan, K.; Trocmé, N.; Jud, A. Child maltreatment-related investigations involving infants: Opportunities for resilience? *Int. J. Child Adolesc. Resielience* **2013**, *1*, 35–47.
17. Herman-Smith, R.; Schmitt, K. Implementing developmental screening programs for infants and toddlers in the child welfare system. *J. Public Child Welf.* **2014**, *8*, 416–432. [CrossRef]
18. Williams, M.E.; Park, S.; Anaya, A.; Perugini, S.M.; Rao, S.; Neece, C.L.; Rafeedie, J. Linking infants and toddlers in foster care to early childhood mental health services. *Child. Youth Serv. Rev.* **2012**, *34*, 838–844. [CrossRef]
19. Berrick, J.D.; Needell, B.; Barth, R.P.; Jonson-Reid, M. *Tender Years: Toward Developmentally Sensitive Child Welfare Services for very Young Children*; Oxford University Press: New York, NY, USA, 1998.
20. Horwitz, S.M.; Hurlburt, M.S.; Heneghan, A.; Zhang, J.; Rolls-Reutz, J.; Landsverk, J.; Stein, R.E.K. Persistence of Mental Health Problems in Very Young Children Investigated by US Child Welfare Agencies. *Acad. Pediatr.* **2013**, *13*, 524–530. [CrossRef] [PubMed]
21. Jones Harden, B. *Infants in the Child Welfare System: A Developmental Framework for Policy and Practice*; Zero To Three: Washington, DC, USA, 2007; ISBN 978-0-943657-97-4.

22. Stahmer, A.C. Developmental and behavioral needs and service use for young children in child welfare. *Pediatrics* **2005**, *116*, 891–900. [CrossRef] [PubMed]

23. Wulczyn, F.; Barth, R.P.; Ying-Ying, T.Y.; Jones Harden, B.; Landsverk, J. *Beyond Common Sense: Child Welfare, Child Well-Being, and the Evidence for Policy Reform*; Transaction Publishers: New Brunswick, NJ, USA, 2005, ISBN 978-0-202-30734-3.

24. Jud, A.; Fallon, B.; Trocmé, N. Who gets services and who does not? Multi-level approach to the decision for ongoing child welfare or referral to specialized services. *Child. Youth Serv. Rev.* **2012**, *34*, 983–988. [CrossRef]

25. Palusci, V.J.; Ondersma, S.J. Services and Recurrence After Psychological Maltreatment Confirmed by Child Protective Services. *Child Maltreat.* **2012**, *17*, 153–163. [CrossRef] [PubMed]

26. Libby, A.M.; Orton, H.D.; Barth, R.P.; Webb, M.B.; Burns, B.J.; Wood, P.; Spicer, P. Alcohol, drug, and mental health specialty treatment services and race/ethnicity: A national study of children and families involved with child welfare. *Am. J. Public Health* **2006**, *96*, 628–631. [CrossRef] [PubMed]

27. Bunger, A.C.; Chuang, E.; McBeath, B. Facilitating mental health service use for caregivers: Referral strategies among child welfare caseworkers. *Child. Youth Serv. Rev.* **2012**, *34*, 696–703. [CrossRef] [PubMed]

28. Filippelli, J.; Fallon, B.; Trocmé, N.; Fuller-Thomson, E.; Black, T. Infants and the decision to provide ongoing child welfare services. *Child Adolesc. Psychiatry Ment. Health* **2017**, *11*, 24. [CrossRef] [PubMed]

29. Connell-Carrick, K. Child abuse and neglect. In *The Wiley Blackwell Handbook of Infant Development*; Bremner, J.G., Wachs, T.D., Eds.; Wiley Blackwell: West Sussex, UK, 2014; pp. 819–845.

30. Johnson, M.R.; Appleyard, K. Infant pychological disorders. In *The Wiley-Blackwell Handbook of Infant Development*; Bremner, J.G., Wachs, T.D., Eds.; John Wiley & Sons: West Sussex, UK, 2014; Volume 1 and 2, pp. 934–961.

31. Dorsey, S.; Kerns, S.E.U.; Trupin, E.W.; Conover, K.L.; Berliner, L. Child welfare caseworkers as service brokers for youth in foster care: Findings from Project Focus. *Child Maltreat.* **2012**, *17*, 22–31. [CrossRef] [PubMed]

32. Kohl, P.L.; Barth, R.P.; Hazen, A.L.; Landsverk, J.A. Child welfare as a gateway to domestic violence services. *Child. Youth Serv. Rev.* **2005**, *27*, 1203–1221. [CrossRef]

33. Hoffman, J.A.; Bunger, A.C.; Robertson, H.A.; Cao, Y.; West, K.Y. Child welfare caseworkers' perspectives on the challenges of addressing mental health problems in early childhood. *Child. Youth Serv. Rev.* **2016**, *65*, 148–155. [CrossRef]

34. Fallon, B.; Ma, J.; Allan, K.; Trocmé, N.; Jud, A. Opportunities for prevention and intervention with young children: Lessons from the Canadian incidence study of reported child abuse and neglect. *Child Adolesc. Psychiatry Ment. Health* **2013**, *7*, 1–13. [CrossRef] [PubMed]

35. Fluke, J.D.; Chabot, M.; Fallon, B.; MacLaurin, B.; Blackstock, C. Placement decisions and disparities among aboriginal groups: An application of the decision making ecology through multi-level analysis. *Child Abuse Negl.* **2010**, *34*, 57–69. [CrossRef] [PubMed]

36. Esposito, T.; Trocmé, N.; Chabot, M.; Shlonsky, A.; Collin-Vézina, D.; Sinha, V. Placement of children in out-of-home care in Québec, Canada: When and for whom initial out-of-home placement is most likely to occur. *Child. Youth Serv. Rev.* **2013**, *35*, 2031–2039. [CrossRef]

37. Fast, E.; Trocmé, N.; Fallon, B.; Ma, J. A troubled group? Adolescents in a Canadian child welfare sample. *Child. Youth Serv. Rev.* **2014**, *46*, 47–54. [CrossRef]

38. Villagrana, M. Pathways to Mental Health Services for Children and Youth in the Child Welfare System: A Focus on Social Workers' Referral. *Child Adolesc. Soc. Work J.* **2010**, *27*, 435–449. [CrossRef]

39. Simmel, C.; Merritt, D.; Kim, S.; Kim, H.M.-S. Developmental Disabilities in Children Involved with Child Welfare: Correlates of Referrals for Service Provision. *J. Public Child Welf.* **2016**, *10*, 197–214. [CrossRef]

40. Johnson-Motoyama, M. Development, CAPTA Part C referral and services among young children in the U.S. child welfare system. *Child Maltreat.* **2016**, *21*, 186–197. [CrossRef] [PubMed]

41. Allen, A.D.; Hyde, J.; Leslie, L.K. "I Don't Know What They Know": Knowledge transfer in mandated referral from child welfare to early intervention. *Child. Youth Serv. Rev.* **2012**, *34*, 1050–1059. [CrossRef]

42. Courtney, M.; Flynn, R.J.; Beaupré, J. Overview of out of home care in the USA and Canada. *Psychosoc. Interv.* **2013**, *22*, 163–173. [CrossRef]

43. Mulcahy, M.; Trocme, N. *Children and Youth in Out-of-Home Care in Canada*; McGill University, Centre for Research on Children and Families: Montreal, QC, Canada, 2010.

44. Trocmé, N.; Kyte, A.; Sinha, V.; Fallon, B. Urgent protection versus chronic need: Clarifying the dual mandate of child welfare services across Canada. *Soc. Sci.* **2014**, *3*, 483–498. [CrossRef]
45. Nikolova, K.; Baird, S.; Tarshis, S.; Black, T.; Fallon, B. Examining the response to different types of exposure to intimate partner violence. *Int. J. Child Adolesc. Resielience* **2014**, *2*, 72–87.
46. Fuller, T. Beyond investigations: differential response in child protective services. In *Handbook of Child Maltreatment*; Springer: New York, NY, USA, 2014; ISBN 978-94-007-7208-3.
47. Wulczyn, F. *Child Well-Being as Human Capital*; Chapin Hall Center for Children at the University of Chicago: Chicago, IL, USA, 2008.
48. Tonmyr, L.; Williams, G.; Jack, S.M.; MacMillan, H.L. Infant placement in Canadian child maltreatment-related investigations. *Int. J. Ment. Health Addict.* **2011**, *9*, 441. [CrossRef]
49. Palusci, V.J. Risk factors and services for child maltreatment among infants and young children. *Child. Youth Serv. Rev.* **2011**, *33*, 1374–1382. [CrossRef]
50. Critical issues in current practice. In *Child Welfare: Connecting Research, Policy, and Practice*; Kufeldt, K.; McKenzie, B. (Eds.) Wilfred Laurier University: Waterloo, ON, Canada, 2011; pp. 553–568.
51. Fallon, B.; Van Wert, M.; Trocmé, N.; MacLaurin, B.; Sinha, V.; Lefebvre, R.; Allan, K.; Black, T. *Ontario Incidence Study of Reported Child Abuse and Neglect-2013 (OIS-2013)*; Canadian Child Welfare Research Portal: Toronto, ON, Canada, 2015.
52. Wright, R.E. Reading and understanding multivariate statistics. In *Reading and Understanding Multivariate Statistics*; American Psychological Association: Washington, DC, USA, 1995; ISBN 978-1-55798-273-5.
53. Bornstein, M.H.; Tamis-LeMonda, C.S. *Wiley-Blackwell Handbook of Infant Development*, 2nd ed.; Wiley-Blackwell: Hoboken, NJ, USA, 2010; Volume 1, pp. 458–482.
54. Fallon, B.; Trocmé, N.; MacLaurin, B. Should child protection services respond differently to maltreatment, risk of maltreatment, and risk of harm? *Child Abuse Negl.* **2011**, *35*, 236–239. [CrossRef] [PubMed]
55. Putnam-Hornstein, E.; Simon, J.; Eastman, A.; Magruder, J. Risk of re-reporting among infants who remain at home following alleged maltreatment. *Child Maltreat.* **2015**, *20*, 92–103. [CrossRef] [PubMed]
56. Hélie, S.; Bouchard, C. Recurrent reporting of child maltreatment: State of knowledge and avenues for research. *Child. Youth Serv. Rev.* **2010**, *32*, 416–422. [CrossRef]
57. Fallon, B.; Ma, J.; Black, T.; Wekerle, C. Characteristics of young parents investigated and opened for ongoing services in child welfare. *Int. J. Ment. Health Addict.* **2011**, *9*, 365–381. [CrossRef]
58. Fallon, B.; Black, T.; Nikolova, K.; Tarshis, S.; Baird, S. Child welfare investigations involving exposure to intimate partner violence: Case and worker characteristics. *Int. J. Child Adolesc. Resielience* **2014**, *2*, 71–76.
59. National Scientific Council on the Developing Child & National Forum on Early Childhood Policy and Programs. *Maternal Depression can Undermine the Development of Young Children*; Harvard University, Center on the Developing Child: Cambridge, MA, USA, 2009.
60. Garland, A.F.; Landsverk, J.A.; Lau, A.S. Racial/ethnic disparities in mental health service use among children in foster care. *Child. Youth Serv. Rev.* **2003**, *25*, 491–507. [CrossRef]
61. Hélie, S. A developmental approach to the risk of a first recurrence in child protective services. *Child Abuse Negl.* **2013**, *37*, 1132–1141. [CrossRef] [PubMed]
62. Baumann, D.J.; Dalgleish, L.; Fluke, J.; Kern, H. *The Decision-Making Ecology*; American Human Association: Washington, DC, USA, 2011.
63. Freisthler, B. Need for and access to supportive services in the child welfare system. *Geoj. Dordr.* **2013**, *78*, 429–441. [CrossRef] [PubMed]
64. Fallon, B.; Trocmé, N. Factors associated with the decision to provide ongoing services: Are worker characteristics and organization geographic location important? In *Child Welfare: Connecting Research, Policy, and Practice*; Kufeldt, K., McKenzie, B., Eds.; Wilfred Laurier University: Waterloo, ON, Canada, 2011; pp. 57–74.
65. Clinton, J.; Kays-Burden, A.; Carter, C.; Bhasin, K.; Cairney, J.; Carrey, N.; Janus, M.; Kulkarni, C.; Williams, R. *Supporting Ontario's Youngest Minds: Investing in the Mental Health of Children under 6*; Ontario Centre of Excellence for Child and Youth Mental Health: Toronto, ON, Canada, 2014.

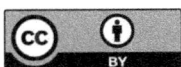

Article

Investing in the Early Childhood Mental Health Workforce Development: Enhancing Professionals' Competencies to Support Emotion and Behavior Regulation in Young Children

Shulamit N. Ritblatt [1],*, Audrey Hokoda [1] and Charles Van Liew [2]

[1] Child and Family Development, San Diego State University, San Diego, CA 92182-4502, USA; audrey.hokoda@mail.sdsu.edu

[2] Humanities Department at Grand Canyon University, Phoenix, AZ 85017, USA; cavanliew@yahoo.com

* Correspondence: ritblatt@mail.sdsu.edu; Tel.: +1-619-594-5312

Received: 28 August 2017; Accepted: 15 September 2017; Published: 19 September 2017

Abstract: This paper delineates a preventive approach to early childhood mental health by preparing the workforce to provide relational, sensitive care to young children ages 0–5. One of the most prevalent issues in early childhood is behavioral challenges and the inability of young children to regulate themselves. This leads to an expulsion rate in early childhood (3–4 times higher than K-12 expulsion rate) and future mental health issues. The Early Childhood Social-Emotional and Behavior Regulation Intervention Specialist (EC-SEBRIS) graduate level certificate program was created to strengthen early care and education providers with the knowledge and practice of how to support emotion and behavior regulation in young children in their groups. Evaluation data provide evidence that early care and education professionals increased in their perception of self-efficacy and in their sensitivity of care and skills to support behavioral health in young children. Results indicated that the children in their care showed less challenging behaviors and increased social competencies. This manuscript highlights the importance of prevention and the dire need to provide young children with high-quality, appropriate care to support their mental health.

Keywords: early childhood; mental health; challenging behaviors; professional training; social emotional development; prevention; early intervention; workforce development

1. Introduction

There are nearly 11 million children under the age of five in the USA whose parents are working while other adults care for them. These children spend an average of 36 h a week in child care and 25% of the children, nearly 3 million, have multiple childcare arrangements as their parents work longer hours and have non-traditional work schedules [1]. As children spend more and more hours in childcare, it becomes increasingly important that early childhood professionals are well educated and trained in recognizing and responding to early signs of social-emotional and mental health problems [2].

Prevalent, serious problems in early childhood include behavioral challenges and the inability to regulate emotions. These behavioral challenges (e.g., aggression, poor self-control, noncompliance, and difficulties socializing with peers) occur in the classrooms of young children once every six minutes [3], and lead to an expulsion rate in preschool settings three to four times higher than K-12 expulsion rates [4,5]. Difficulties regulating emotions and behaviors are associated with internalizing and externalizing behavioral problems in young children that may result in lifelong psychiatric disorders and maladjustments [6–8]. For example, poor emotion regulation is associated with depression, anxiety, schizophrenia, and post-traumatic stress disorder [9–11], sexual promiscuity [12], and physical health issues [13–15]. If left untreated, young children with challenging behavior are more likely to display at-risk behaviors as adolescents, such as delinquency, gang involvement, and substance abuse; in fact, early childhood behavior problems are the single best predictor for several of these long-term outcomes [16].

Emotional and behavioral regulation in young children is critical to healthy mental development and research suggests that this regulatory skill is acquired via emotionally attuned adult–child interactions. In the absence of these interactions, the ability to regulate emotion is impaired as well as the architecture of the developing brain [17,18]. Early positive experiences support the creation of circuits in the brain that are responsible for generating emotions, behavioral responses, perception, and bodily sensations [19]. Studies have documented the impact of early childhood stress (e.g., adverse childhood experiences) on neurobiological development that has long-term effects on anxiety, aggression, self-regulation, cognition, and social-emotional functioning (e.g., [20,21]).

Growing evidence suggests that the prevention and early intervention are needed particularly for young children who experience prolonged toxic stress. Research also demonstrates that, when early childhood stress is experienced, stable supportive relationships with adults can buffer these harmful effects and facilitate adaptive coping responses. "To that end, there is a critical need for creative new interventions that strengthen the capacity of parents and other caregivers to reduce sources of excessive adversity and to help build effective coping skills in children who experience high levels of stress" [22] (p. 1645).

The purpose of this paper is (a) to highlight research emphasizing the critical role of adult–child relationships as the foundation of mental health and a buffer to negative experiences and toxic stress; (b) to describe a training model (Early Childhood Social Emotional and Behavior Regulation Intervention Specialist, EC-SEBRIS, program), a preventive approach to early childhood mental health that prepares the workforce to provide relational, sensitive care to young children ages 0–5; and (c) to provide outcome data indicating the effects of the training on the early childhood professionals participating in the year-long program and the children they served.

1.1. The Importance of Adult–Child Relationships and Early Childhood Care and Education in Promoting Mental Health

An abundance of translational, cross-disciplinary studies (e.g., [23]) have helped us understand young children's development and mental health are outcomes of an ongoing interaction between nature and nurturer [24,25]. This biodevelopmental approach [26] recognizes the link between emotion, the brain, and the body, and highlights the importance of positive interactions and stable relationships in meeting the specific developmental needs of the young child [27–31].

Poor quality of care in early years is a major contributor to toxic stress [32]. Continuous elevated levels of the stress hormone, cortisol, have permanent negative changes on the brain [33]. Research findings [34,35] provide support for the notion that sensitive and responsive caregiving helps children express distress without elevating cortisol levels while anticipating adults' help.

A critical piece of the puzzle in providing high quality relationships lies with the early childhood teachers with whom many children spend a majority of their time. It takes one caring adult who has a positive relationship with a child to protect the child, especially those children who experience multiple risks and stressors [36]. These positive out-of-home relationships can change the attachment internal working models developed by the children with their parents and buffer them from the risks of adverse caregiving received in the home [37].

Multiple studies have been conducted on teacher–child relationships and the results point to the overwhelmingly positive and lasting effects of close teacher–child relationships on children emotionally, socially, and academically [38–45]. For example, positive sensitive teacher–child relationships appear to decrease behavioral challenges and the negative effects for children at risk for externalizing and internalizing problems [38,46]. Similarly, numerous studies on positive behavior support in early childhood education settings indicate that effective behavior management in the classrooms support young children's abilities to regulate their emotions and behaviors and yield better child outcomes [47–50].

It is important to understand that the stress, burnout, and frustration early childhood educators feel in their jobs affect their relationships with the children in their care and the environments they create for the children. Educators who experience a high level of stress are less likely to engage in warm, responsive caregiving and experience more negative behaviors in the classroom [51,52]. Early childhood professionals point out that dealing with challenging behaviors is their number one stressor, and teachers also report feeling unprepared to support emotion and behavior regulation and that they experience a high level of frustration and helplessness on a daily basis.

An effective way to enhance early childhood professionals' capacity to provide warm, responsive caregiving and reduce problem behaviors and rates of expulsion is giving professionals greater access to mental health consultation [5,53–55]. Unfortunately, only 23% of teachers in an early childhood settings report regular access to a mental health consultant [56]. Furthermore, more frequent consultations are associated with lower turnover of teachers, improved effectiveness of teachers, and an enhanced program quality [53,57,58]. Research further indicates that, when mental health consultants are housed within the early childhood education programs, they are found to be more effective in their work with children and teachers [59–62]. In addition to mental health consultation, it is recommended that reflective practice is included in educational programs and trainings for caregivers and early childhood educators [63]. Insightfulness is critical to the understanding of the child's internal world, enhances caregivers' sensitivity, and facilitates the development of secure attachments [64–67].

The research presented above shows that early experiences have long-lasting effects on the developmental trajectory of the child and their mental health, and that nurturing, sensitive, and responsive relationships between adults and young children are critical in ensuring the provision of high-quality care [22]. Prevention and early intervention is needed particularly for young children who experience adversity and toxic stress [22], and quality early childhood care and education can serve as a buffer and promote healthy mental development in young children. Specifically, professional training that focuses on emotional and behavior regulation support is essential for early childhood professionals working with young children [68]. The following section describes an innovative, cutting-edge training program designed to prepare a workforce of early childhood professionals to provide sensitive relational care and to address early mental health problems with behavior and emotional regulation.

1.2. Training Model: Early Childhood Social Emotional and Behavior Regulation Intervention Specialist (EC-SEBRIS) Program

The underlying assumption that has guided the development and implementation of the Early Childhood Social-Emotional and Behavior Regulation Intervention Specialist (EC-SEBRIS) Certificate Program ([69] is that the early childhood professional is an important member of the first-response "mental health" team to manage children's needs and daily care. The EC-SEBRIS was designed to help teachers and early childhood professionals develop the skills and competencies needed to address challenging behaviors in their classrooms or at homes, so that they can meet the critical social-emotional and behavioral needs of young children.

Therefore, the purpose of the EC-SEBRIS Certificate Program is to establish a recognition and response model to meet the needs of increasing numbers of young children who attend childcare programs and have social-emotional and behavioral challenges and to help early childhood professionals be more self-aware and emotionally available to provide the children under their care with sensitive, warm, and responsive positive interactions. The program is based on the Teaching Pyramid (National Center in the Social and Emotional Foundations for Early Learning—CSEFEL), and has three levels of training teachers to address emotional and behavioral problems among young children. The first level—*Promotion (Tier I)*—a prevention approach that targets children who are at risk of poor developmental outcomes, including early identification using screenings and improving the quality of child care (ages 0–5) that encourages brain development, learning, and emotional well-being of all young children. The second level—*Preventive Intervention (Tier 2)*—targets children who already exhibit emotional and behavioral problems and provides them and their families with highly specialized levels of service that mitigate the effects of risk and stress and address potential early relationship challenges or vulnerabilities that affect early development. The third level—*Treatment (Tier 3)*—targets children in distress or with clear symptoms indicating mental health disorder to provide them and their families with highly specialized levels of service by skilled staff [68].

The EC-SEBRIS Certificate Program targets early childhood professionals (i.e., students) in the field who have earned an undergraduate degree in Child Development or related areas. Following the recommendations described in the Delivery of Infant-Family and Early Mental Health Services Training Guidelines and Personnel Competencies proposed by California's Infant, Preschool and Family Mental Health Initiative (2010), it uses a wraparound triple method of teaching that includes three main domains: Knowledge, Experience, and Reflective Supervision (see Figure 1).

As depicted in Figure 1, the *Knowledge* domain is covered in 4 seminar courses (over the course of two consecutive semesters): (1) Seminar in Child Development Theories-Intervention and Prevention, which reviews attachment and affect regulation theories, assessment, and screening information for differentiating typical and atypical development in young children (0–5) and strategies for implementing a regulation plan at childcare sites; (2) Seminar in Human Development: Positive Behavior Support for Young Children with Challenging Behavior, which teaches students how to implement best practice interventions that promote social-emotional and behavioral development in young children (0–5); (3) Eco-behavioral Assessment and Intervention, which reviews eco-behavioral assessment techniques (e.g., direct observations, rating scales, structured interviews, analogue measures) and behavior analytic intervention strategies promoting social-behavioral development; and (4) Advanced Applied Behavior Analysis, which reviews Applied Behavior Analysis (ABA) with a focus on teaching positive social interaction and self-management skills to young children.

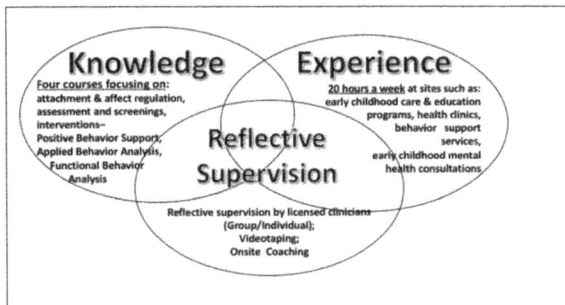

Figure 1. Early Childhood Social Emotional and Behavior Regulation Intervention Specialist (EC-SEBRIS) Certificate Triple Mode Teaching Model.

As part of the *Experience* Domain, students were required to work a minimum of 20 h a week providing direct services/education to children 0–5 years of age. The majority of the students enrolled in the program had a job in which they provided direct service/education to children of this age group. These work sites were considered as the students' practicum sites where they could apply and practice the knowledge and skills learned in their courses. The underlying notion was that the application of knowledge at the same site that the student spent most of their time working with young children can benefit the children and can have a ripple effect on the other providers at the site. The sites included early childhood education programs, agencies providing mental health and behavior support services, home visitation programs, and others.

The *Reflective Supervision* domain includes the following components: reflective facilitation for students (group and individual), video feedback, and on-site coaching. This triple method of coaching and mentoring supports the reflective process and provides the student with an opportunity to identify their own needs and potential areas of growth [70–72]. According to The California Infant, Preschool and Family Mental Health Initiative: Training Guidelines and Recommended Personnel Competencies [73], reflective supervision is essential when working with young children. Research suggested that it can enhance caregivers' sensitivity. Hence, experienced licensed clinical supervisors provided bi-monthly individual supervision and weekly group supervision. During group supervision, students practice concepts and theoretical information presented in the foundation courses. Students "learn by doing" and by discussing their experiences using their video recordings with other students [63].

As mentioned above, students in the EC-SEBRIS Certificate Program were equipped with a video camera and were asked to videotape their interactions with children once a week for 30–45 min. Videotaping of teacher–child interactions has been found to support the reflective process needed for the adult to be more aware and sensitive when interacting with young children [74]. Viewing these recordings with their peers and the clinical reflective supervisor provided students the opportunity to "see" themselves as they interact with children and be aware of the transactional nature of their interactions with the children.

The Reflective Supervision domain included on-site coaching [75–77]. The coaches were highly experienced early childhood intervention professionals who have had extensive experience working with children, families and other professionals in the early childhood intervention and education field. The visits of onsite coaches took place four to five times a year (two to three times each semester). These coaches assisted students in assessing their initial skills level and establishing goals and objectives for future professional growth and self-improvement.

1.3. Evaluation of EC-SEBRIS Program

A third goal of this paper is to present outcome data evaluating the effects of the training on the early childhood professionals who graduated from the program and the children they served. Specifically, this study examines the following questions: (1) Did the students enrolled in EC-SEBRIS Certificate Program show an increase in their ability to provide sensitive, responsive care and support behavioral and emotional regulation in young children? (2) Did children improve in their social-emotional functioning after the intervention was offered to them by the students as reported by parents?

2. Materials and Methods

This study evaluates the effectiveness of the Early Childhood Social-Emotional and Behavior Regulation Intervention Specialist (EC-SEBRIS) Certificate Program. Questions focus on whether the students enrolled in the program show an increase in their ability to offer sensitive, responsive care, provide behavior support, and promote social emotional development, and whether the children improved in behavior and emotion regulation after the students worked with them. The study used mixed methods (observations, surveys) and multiple sources (students, site supervisors, parents).

2.1. Participants

2.1.1. Students

The sample consisted of 154 individuals (93.51% female; 6.49% male). The age group distribution of the sample was 46.10% were between 18 and 24 years, 22.73% were between 25 and 29 years, 15.58% were between 30 and 39 years, 8.44% were between 40 and 49 years, 5.19% were between 50 and 59 years, and 1.95% were 60 years or older. Ethnically, 45.45% identified as White, 35.71% identified as Hispanic, 8.44% identified as Black, 4.55% identified as Asian or Pacific Islander, 2.6% identified as Middle Eastern, and 3.25% identified as multi-ethnic. Ninety-five students were monolingual and 59 students were at least bilingual. English was the most common primary language (72.08%), followed by Spanish (21.43%) and other (6.49%).

The evaluation of the EC-SEBRIS certificate program started with the 2nd Cohort and proceeded into a more comprehensive evaluation with the third Cohort, hence the evaluation focused on 4–5 cohorts. 22 to 35 students graduated each year from the certificate program. Demographics of the cohorts under evaluation (see Table 1) indicate that there were no significant differences among these cohorts in these domains per analyses.

Table 1. Participant Demographics.

Item	Cohort 0		Cohort 1		Cohort 2		Cohort 3		Cohort 4	
	Valid %	N	Valid %	N	Valid %	N	Valid %	N	Valid %	N
Ethnicity										
White	44.44	12	48.6	17	32.0	8	57.6	19	41.7	10
Hispanic	40.74	11	22.9	8	48.0	12	30.3	10	37.5	9
Black	7.41	2	11.4	4	-	-	-	-	4.2	1
Other	7.41	2	17.2	6	20.0	5	12.1	4	16.7	4
Undergraduate Major										
Child and Family	40.74	11	48.3	17	48.0	12	48.5	16	62.5	15
Social Science (Other)	14.81	4	31.4	11	36.0	9	33.3	11	25.0	6
Language	14.81	4	5.7	2	-	-	9.1	3	-	-
Communication or Arts	11.11	3	-	-	-	-	6.1	2	4.2	1
Other	18.52	5	14.3	5	16.0	4	3.0	1	8.3	2
Mental Health Experience										
Yes	18.52	5	18.2	6	20.0	5	21.2	7	45.8	11
No	81.48	22	81.8	27	80.0	20	78.8	26	54.2	13
Bilingual										
Yes	18.52	5	37.1	13	60.0	15	33.3	11	27.5	9
No	81.48	22	62.9	22	40.0	10	66.7	22	62.5	15
Primary Language										
English	85.19	23	62.9	22	56.0	14	75.8	25	87.5	21
Spanish	14.81	4	20.0	7	32.0	8	24.2	8	8.3	2
Other	-	-	17.1	6	12.0	3	-	-	4.2	1
Second Language										
English	-	-	100	13	66.7	10	72.7	8	33.3	3
Spanish	80.0	4	-	-	13.3	2	18.2	2	55.6	5
Other	20.0	1	-	-	20.0	3	9.1	1	11.1	1

2.1.2. Supervisors

Sixty-four (64) supervisors of students enrolled in the certificate program were asked to complete surveys assessing the competencies of students and how the student's enrollment in the EC-SEBRIS Certificate Program affected their practicum site. The students worked as master teachers in preschools, behavioral health specialists, home visitors, early interventionists, special educators, and directors of agencies. The supervisors were asked to complete a survey at the beginning of the first semester (September/October) and at the end of the second semester (April/May).

2.1.3. Parents

Parents of children at students' practicum sites whose child received behavior regulation support from the student were asked to rate their children's social competencies and behavioral challenges prior to the start of the intervention (pre- at the beginning of the first semester, October–November) and then respond again to the survey at the end of the second semester (post-April–May). Sixty-three (63) parents completed a pre-post survey about the emotional and social skills of their child. The lower number of parent respondents is due to the transient nature of children placed in early childhood setting or coming to services. Often, a student would start working with a specific child in the fall and had to switch and work with another child in the spring. This means that the pre-survey done in the fall did not match the post-survey done in the spring by another parent of a different child. Hence, the total number of matching pre-post is 63.

2.2. Measures

2.2.1. The Caregiver Interaction Scale (CIS)

Quality of care provided by early childhood professionals was measured using The Arnett Caregiver Interaction Scale (CIS) [78]. This tool measures the verbal and physical interactions between the providers and the children in their classrooms. It is designed for use during observation of teacher caregiving skills. The CIS contains 26 items, categorized into four subscales: teacher sensitivity (10 items), harshness (9 items), detachment (4 items), and permissiveness (3 items) towards children [79]. Items on this scale are rated on a 4-point scale of *Not at All, Somewhat, Quite a Bit, and Most of the Time* [79]. These items are grouped into the four subscales and mean scores are calculated to determine caregiver interactions [80].

To assess the level of sensitivity and positive interactions which are critical to mental health, observations were performed to determine whether there were changes in sensitivity amongst students' overtime based on scores collected from the CIS, specifically in the area of measure categorized as "sensitivity". The sensitivity section of the CIS examines whether or not the student, "speaks warmly to the children", "listens attentively when children speak to her", "seems to enjoy the children", "when the children misbehave, explains the reason for the rule they are breaking", "encourages the children to try new experiences", "seems enthusiastic about the children's activities and efforts", "pays positive attention to the children as individuals", "talks to children on a level they can understand", "encourages children to exhibit prosocial behavior, e.g., sharing, helping", and "when talking to children, kneels, bends, or sits at their level to establish better eye contact". The Arnett Caregiver Interaction Scale was internally consistent, with Cronbach's $\alpha = 0.85$ and 0.86 at baseline and follow-up, respectively.

2.2.2. Supervisor Survey

This 10-item Likert-scale survey ask supervisors how the student's enrollment in the EC-SEBRIS Certificate Program has impacted the practicum site (e.g., childcare center, behavioral services, or kindergarten classroom). The pre-post scale provides an opportunity for the supervisor to rank the student on a scale from 1 to 4 (1 = Strongly disagree; 2 = Disagree; 3 = Agree; 4 = Strongly agree) on the areas of knowledge and experience that the students in the program are believed to be focusing on in their classes and reflective supervision. The supervisor survey was developed partially following the Goal Achievement Scale (GAS)-ECE Center Director [57]. The GAS tool was administered to child care directors and teachers to measure teachers' competencies on general mental health activities or program goals. The supervisor survey includes 10 items such as "Student understands children's social and emotional development"; "Student tries to understand the meaning of children's behavior"; "Student is able to manage children's challenging behaviors"; "Student responds appropriately and effectively to children in distress"; "Student is capable of reflecting on experiences, thoughts and feelings involved in working with infants, young children and families". The supervisor survey also exhibited good internal reliability, with Cronbach's $\alpha = 0.91$ and 0.91 at baseline and follow-up, respectively.

2.2.3. Self-Efficacy (SE) Survey

A self-efficacy measure assessing students' confidence in achieving the evidence-based competencies for promoting social and emotional development and addressing challenging behavior in young children (described by the National Center on the Social and Emotional Foundations for Early Learning; CSEFEL) was used. The EC-SEBRIS faculty worked on this tool during the first year of the program to adapt the tool to match the targeted competencies and foci of the EC-SEBRIS certificate objectives. In this measure, students were asked to rate how confident they are in their ability to use promotion, prevention, and intervention levels of competencies to support young children's social and emotional development. Students rate their abilities to develop nurturing and responsive relationships, create high quality environments, provide targeted social emotional supports, and implement intensive interventions. Each of these four general areas includes items relating to knowledge, skills, and reflective practice that promote social emotional competence in young children.

The survey has 60 items needed to be rated on a Likert scale of 1–5 (1 = Not at all confident; 2 = A little confident; 3 = Somewhat confident; 4 = Fairly confident; and 5 = Very confident).

The Nurturing and Responsive Relationships (NRR) domain is comprised of 24 items (1–24) focusing on the quality of the relationships formed with the child and their family (Tier 1). The following is a list sample items from this domain: "Develop meaningful relationships with children and families"; "Use a variety of strategies for building relationships with all families"; "Withhold judgment and feel empathy for parent/caregiver's perspectives"; "Help parents/caregivers to appreciate the uniqueness of their young child"; "Show sensitivity to individual children's needs and adapt and adjust accordingly (instruction, curriculum, materials, etc.)"; "Assess children's strengths across all developmental and behavioral dimensions"; "Practice responsive caregiving based on the understanding each child's unique development, responding to the child's cues and signals, and following the child's lead"; "Model appropriate expressions, labeling children's emotions, and self-regulation".

High Quality Environment (HQE) is the second domain in this survey (Tier 1). It consists of 19 items (25–43) addressing such issues as: "Asses children's development and learning, including cognitive and language skills, social emotional development, approaches to learning, and health and physical development"; "Observe and document children's work, play behaviors and interactions to assess progress"; "Manage behaviors and implement classroom rules and expectations in a manner that is consistent and predictable"; "Design activities to promote engagement (e.g., varies topics and activities in large and small groups from day to day, varies speech intonation to maintain children's interest; modifies plans when children lose interest uses peers as models)"; "Provides children with varied opportunities to learn to understand, empathize with, and take into account other's people perspectives"; "Teach staff to support children's development of friendships and provide opportunities for children to play and learn from each other".

Social Emotional Support (SES) is the third domain in the Self-Efficacy survey and addresses the promotion of prosocial behaviors and social emotional skills (Tier 1). There are (44–52) nine (9) items, which include the following: "Help children talk about their own and others' emotions"; Provide children with varied opportunities to develop skills for entering into social groups, developing friendships, learning to help, and other pro-social behavior"; "Establishes and enforce clear rules, limits, and consequences for behavior"; "Teach staff to assist children in resolving conflicts by helping them identify feelings, describe problems, and try alternative solutions".

The last domain in the survey is Intensive Interventions (II). This domain includes 8 items (53–60) addressing the ability to provide intervention to children who exhibit challenging behaviors (Tiers 2 and 3). For example, students were asked to rate their ability to "Team with a family to develop support plans for intensive interventions"; "Assess the presence and extent of atypical child behavior that may be a barrier to intervention and progress"; "Work as a team to develop and implement an individualized plan that supports inclusion and success with children with persistent, serious, challenging behavior"; "Assess problem behaviors in context to identify its function, and then devise interventions that are comprehensive in that they make the problem behavior irrelevant, inefficient, and ineffective". The Self-Efficacy scales had very high internal reliability, with Cronbach's $\alpha = 0.95$, 0.96, 0.93, and 0.94 for NRR, HQE, SES, and II at baseline and Cronbach's $\alpha = 0.93$, 0.96, 0.93, and 0.92 at follow-up.

2.2.4. Parent Survey

A Likert-scale survey was developed for parents, whose child received intervention, a targeted individualized behavior regulation plan, throughout their time in the EC-SEBRIS Certificate Program, to report the perceived change in their child. The survey consisted of items following the Desired Results Developmental Profile (DRDP) standards for social emotional development. Parents were asked to rate their child's social competencies and behavioral challenges to determine whether their children were impacted from the students' enrollment in the EC-SEBRIS Certificate Program, once in the beginning of the first semester and once at the end of the second semester (pre/post). The Likert 12-item scale has 4 levels of responses: 1 = Strongly disagree; 2 = Disagree; 3 = Agree; and 4 = Strongly agree. For example, parents were asked to indicate if they agree with the following: "Child understands that own physical characteristics and preferences are separate from others"; "Child shows awareness of other's feelings and responds to other's feelings appropriate"; "Child uses socially appropriate ways to stop self from acting impulsively"; "Child develops understanding of taking turns"; Child interacts cooperatively with other children through play"; Child forms friendships with other children"; "Child learns to understand the needs of other children and tries to follow social rules". The parent survey had good internal consistency, with Cronbach's α = 0.90 and 0.88 at baseline and follow-up, respectively.

2.3. Procedure

Human Subjects approval was granted following the review of the research protocol to the EC-SEBRIS certificate program. All participants (students, parents, and supervisors) were given a consent form to sign prior to their participation in the evaluation process.

Incoming students, during an orientation retreat in the summer, were informed about the program and its evaluation process and were given a consent form to sign in order to participate in the evaluation process of the program. The voluntary participation in this study was emphasized. Therefore, students were aware that the decision of whether or not to participate would not influence their future relations with or status in the certificate program. Certificate students were assured that their grades would not be affected by their decision to participate. In addition, students were informed that they are free to withdraw consent and to discontinue participation at any time without penalty or loss of benefits.

Confidentiality was maintained by removing personal information on the surveys. Instead numerical codes were given so pre- and post-scores could be matched without the need to identify the student. All surveys were kept in a locked cabinet in a locked room and were available only to the SDSU program evaluators.

Self-Efficacy survey was administered twice (pre–post) at the beginning of the program (August/September) and then at the end of the program (April/May). Supervisor surveys were self-administered to the supervisors at the beginning of fall semester and at the end of spring semester. Parent surveys were administered in the beginning of the school year and once at the end of the school year. Parents were given the surveys and completed them at home. They returned the survey in a sealed envelope.

Observations using the Arnett Caregiver Interaction Scale were administered by a trained evaluator. The evaluator/observer was trained to use the scale and was compared to faculty and other students trained to use it as well. Training was extensive and lasted until the inter-rater agreement reached 80%. Initial observations took place from September to November and the follow-up observation took place towards the end of the program (March–May). Observations took place at students' work/volunteer sites while they interacted with the child/children for whom they were creating a regulation, prevention and/or intervention plan.

3. Results

In order to understand the results, it is important to clarify that the evaluation process started a year following the implementation of the program. Each cohort, as presented in Table 2 (Demographics by Cohort), was comprised of 22–35 students whose ethnicity, undergraduate major, and mental health experience contributed to the similarities and differences among the cohorts. For example, 48% of Cohort 2's students were Hispanic, compared with only 22.9% in Cohort 1; 62.5% of the students in Cohort 4 had Child and Family as their undergraduate major, while around 48% of students from the other Cohorts earned their undergraduate degree majoring in Child and Family; 48% of students in Cohort 4 indicated having experience in mental health vs. only 18–21% of students in the other Cohorts. The evaluation of the EC-SEBRIS focused on the changes measured in the pre- and post-observations and survey reports; however, analyses were performed considering the possibility of differences between cohorts, which were independent groups. Analyses were performed with full factorial models, including the interaction of Cohort by Time (pre-post). However, with respect to the primary purposes of this paper, the main effect of Time was of principal interest.

Table 2. The Effects of Time, Cohort, and Time × Cohort on Arnett Caregiver Interaction Scale (CIS).

	F (dfd = 113)	p	R^2	M Pre/Post
Quality				
Time (dfn = 1)	67.12	<0.001	0.373	
Cohort (dfn = 3)	6.7.9	<0.001	0.153	3.15/3.35
Time × Cohort (dfn = 3)	0.35	0.786	0.009	
Sensitivity				
Time (dfn = 1)	98.57	<0.001	0.466	
Cohort (dfn = 3)	75.61	<0.001	0.667	2.59/2.95
Time × Cohort (dfn = 3)	0.25	0.863	0.023	
Harshness				
Time (dfn = 1)	2.34	0.128	0.005	
Cohort (dfn = 3)	45.68	<0.001	0.474	1.25/1.20
Time × Cohort (dfn = 3)	2.97	0.035	0.023	
Detachment				
Time (dfn = 1)	30.81	<0.001	0.214	
Cohort (dfn = 3)	9.49	<0.001	0.201	3.51/3.76
Time × Cohort (dfn = 3)	0.41	0.744	0.011	
Permissiveness				
Time (dfn = 1)	1.48	0.226	0.013	
Cohort (dfn = 3)	151.64	<0.001	0.801	2.97/3.01
Time × Cohort (dfn = 3)	9.75	<0.001	0.206	

dfd = degree of freedom in the denominator; dfn = degree of freedom in the nominator.

3.1. Question 1

Did the students enrolled in EC-SEBRIS Certificate Program show an increase in their ability to provide sensitive, responsive care and support behavioral and emotional regulation in young children?

3.1.1. Effects of Training on Students' Competencies

Three sources of data were used in order to answer this question: direct pre-post observation of the students using the Arnett Scale, pre-post surveys of the site directors, and students' pre-post self-efficacy report.

3.1.2. Arnett Caregiver Interaction Scale (CIS)

A series of mixed-effects Analysis of Variance analysis, ANOVAs nesting students within cohorts were performed to assess the effects of Time and Cohort (1–4) on CIS scores. There were significant effects of Cohort on every scale. More importantly, results showed significant main effects of Time on Quality, Sensitivity, and Detachment. Additionally, there were significant interactions of Time by Cohort on Harshness and Permissiveness (see Table 2).

3.1.3. Supervisor and Director Surveys on Student's Performance

A mixed-effects hierarchical linear model was performed to assess the effects of Time and Cohort (1–4) on mean Supervisor Evaluations, where student was nested as a random factor within Cohort and supervisor was specified as a secondary random factor. There were 64 supervisors to 100 students with the average supervisor rating 2 students, and the maximum number of ratings from a single supervisor was 23. Models were performed with and without the interaction and compared using the $\Delta\chi^2$ test to determine whether the interaction significantly improved the model. The $\Delta\chi^2(3) = 0.62$, $p = 0.892$ demonstrated that the pithier model without the interaction was statistically superior; therefore, it was interpreted. The model was significant, Wald $\chi^2(4, N = 139) = 25.42$, $p < 0.001$. There was also a significant main effect of Time, $B = 0.179$, $z = 3.46$, $p = 0.001$, demonstrating that students received higher evaluations post-program.

Supervisors in their comments indicated that students improved in their knowledge and skills supporting children's development and dealing with challenging behaviors: "The EC-SEBRIS student showed lots of growth during his time here. His biggest area of growth was building relationships with parents and caregivers"; "I feel that the student gained experience working directly with families, teachers and children. She excelled in building bonds with parents as her role was to meet with them, provide resources, and create goals"; "The student has a much stronger understanding of social emotional development and is a more competent parent educator, specifically for in-home behavioral support services"; and, "The student has grown exponential. She started the year out with infants and did such an amazing job. She really tuned into the children and their needs and has such a gentle and caring demeanor with them".

3.1.4. Self-Efficacy (SE)-Student's Self Report

A series of mixed-effect ANOVAs nesting students within cohorts were performed to assess the effects of Time and Cohort (0–4) on mean SE domains. The effect of Time was significant on all subscales of the SE measure, as well as the Total (see Table 3). Although there were significant interactions of Cohort by Time for most scales and the Total (see Figure 2), these interactions were quantitative in nature, meaning some cohorts improved slightly more than others, although all cohorts improved.

The effect of Time was significant on all subscales of the SE measure, as well as Total; $F(1, 270) = 415.42$, $p < 0.001$, and Cohort, $F(4, 270) = 9.71$, $p < 0.001$, and a significant interaction, $F(4, 270) = 3.73$, $p = 0.006$ (see Figure 2). The effect of Time demonstrated that averaged across Cohort, SE Total increased from Pre- (M = 3.38) to Post-Program (M = 4.66) (see Table 3).

Table 3. The Effects of Time, Cohort, and Time $\times$ Cohort on Self-Efficacy.

	F (dfd = 135)	p	R^2	M Pre/Post
SE NRR				
Time (dfn = 1)	413.11	<0.001	0.754	
Cohort (dfn = 4)	9.10	<0.001	0.212	3.55/4.67
Time $\times$ Cohort (dfn = 4)	5.13	<0.001	0.132	
SE HQE				
Time (dfn = 1)	398.63	<0.001	0.747	
Cohort (dfn = 4)	6.84	<0.001	0.169	3.41/4.67
Time $\times$ Cohort (dfn = 4)	4.54	0.002	0.119	
SE SES				
Time (dfn = 1)	342.68	<0.001	0.717	
Cohort (dfn = 4)	6.02	<0.001	0.151	3.46/4.72
Time $\times$ Cohort (dfn = 4)	3.81	0.006	0.101	
SE II				
Time	465.97	<0.001	0.775	
Cohort	3.52	0.009	0.094	2.75/4.53
Time $\times$ Cohort	1.58	0.18	0.045	
SE Total				
Time (dfn = 1)	493.71	<0.001	0.785	
Cohort (dfn = 4)	8.38	<0.001	0.199	3.38/4.66
Time $\times$ Cohort (dfn = 4)	4.44	0.002	0.116	

Note: dfd = degree of freedom in the denominator; dfn = degree of freedom in the nominator; SE = Self-Efficacy; NRR = Nurturing and Responsive Relationships; HQE = High Quality Environment; SES = Social Emotional Support; II = Intensive Interventions.

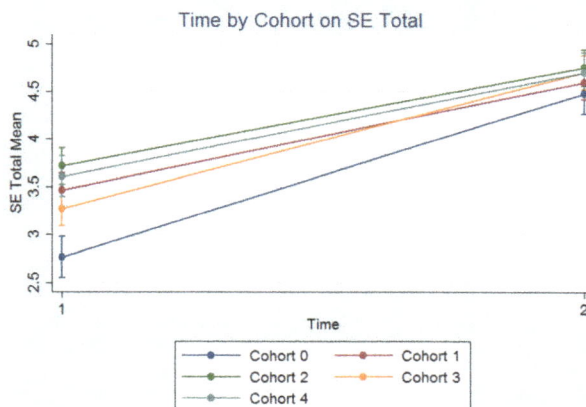

Figure 2. The Effects of Time and Cohort on Self Efficacy (SE) Total Scores.

Although the Cohorts did differ from one another on the SE measures averaged across time, results indicate that students enrolled in the EC-SEBRIS certificate program in all cohorts have increased in their self-efficacy. Any interactions that existed were quantitative in nature, indicating that some Cohorts experienced greater increases in self-efficacy than others, but all increased. Students perceived themselves at the end of the program as better able to develop meaningful relationships with children and their families, to interact and respond sensitively to children meeting their needs, to create a safe environment where children's needs are met, to partner and work with families respecting their cultural beliefs, to assess, observe, document, and design activities and interactions that can promote the child's social emotional skills, to structure routines and provide environments where the child can engage, interact, communicate, learn, and feel competent, and to help children to socialize and interact with peers and other adults.

Overall, all Self Efficacy (SE) measures showed significant improvement across the duration of the program averaged across all cohorts.

3.2. Question 2

Did children improve in their social-emotional functioning after the intervention was offered to them by the students as reported by parents?

Parent Surveys on Child's Social Emotional Skills

A mixed-effects ANOVA was performed to assess the effects of and Cohort (1–4) on mean Parent Survey scores. Results showed a significant main effect of Time, $F(1, 113) = 10.03$, $p = 0.002$, but no effect of Cohort, $F(3, 113) = 0.98$, $p = 0.405$, or the interaction, $F(3, 113) = 0.91$, $p = 0.440$. The effect of Time demonstrated that across all cohorts parents provided higher evaluations at Post-Program (M = 3.25) than Pre-Program (M = 3.01).

Parents recognized the improvement in their child's social competencies and behaviors. Parents indicated that their child was able to regulate their emotions and behaviors, stopped biting, started using their words, had fewer tantrums, and were able to use social skills to befriend the children around them. Some examples of comments from parents are as follows: "My child has made a lot of progress from the pre-survey. For example, I have noticed that she shares toys with others and asks other children if she can borrow toys from them. Additionally, I am noticing that she is more familiar with emotions"; "I have noticed that he is able to calm himself down when he became frustrated or upset. He verbalizes his emotions and is able to name his feelings. He is aware that he has the ability to calm himself down, leading to more cooperative interactions"; "My child is literally a different person! She has become less violent and more compassionate towards other people. Prior to this program, my daughter had no friends and other kids were afraid of her. Now, she has friends and the kids actually want to play with her".

4. Discussion

This paper describes a preventive approach to early childhood mental health with a focus on a professional development program (EC-SEBRIS) that prepares a workforce of early childhood professionals to provide relational sensitive care and to support emotion and behavior regulation in young children. Behavioral challenges occur often in classrooms, lead to high preschool expulsion rates, and can lead to long-term mental health problems. This primary prevention approach targets children and their families before an intervention is needed as it equips ECE professionals who work with young children on a daily basis with the skills and competencies to support children's healthy development, address problem behaviors on-site, and provide them with a safe, familiar adult who is able to "contain" their frustrations and temperaments and help them learn effective coping skills to handle stress.

The EC-SEBRIS program addresses a vital need that early childhood professionals be trained to recognize and respond to early signs of social-emotional and mental health problems [2]. The program uses a wraparound triple method of teaching recommendations for infant family and early mental health services [73] that includes core content coursework, practicum experiences, and reflective supervision. Core content coursework is focused on attachment and affect regulation theories, assessment, and screening for typical and atypical development, as well as best practices of intervention strategies (e.g., Positive Behavior Support- PBS, Applied Behavior Analysis-ABA) that can help mitigate the effects of stress and address emotional and behavioral challenges in young children. Practicum experiences involved 20 h a week providing direct services/education to young children, and since most of the students had direct service jobs, their practicum classes allowed them to apply the knowledge and skills learned in their coursework to current behavioral problems and challenges they faced at their workplace. The EC-SEBRIS also followed recommendations that training of early childhood professionals include greater access to mental health consultation and reflective supervision [5,53–55,63] as the program included individual and group sessions with a licensed mental health professional, and use of videotaping and on-site coaching to further students' abilities to address social-emotional and behavioral challenges in young children.

This study provides support that the EC-SEBRIS program was successful in promoting positive outcomes for the ECE professionals (students) enrolled in the program and for the children and families they served. Observations of students interacting with young children at their practicum sites indicate that the students increased in Sensitivity scores on the Arnett Caregiver Interaction Scale. That is, they appeared to have improved in their positive interactions with children: speaking more warmly to them, listening attentively, and enjoying being with them. The results provide evidence that the students increased in behaviors that encouraged children to explore, learn new things, and exhibit prosocial behaviors.

Further evidence that the students increased in their abilities to provide behavior support and enhance social emotional development in young children is provided by surveys given to their site supervisor. Analyses of scores on the Goal Achievement Scale for supervisors revealed that students improved on teaching competencies that include a greater understanding of children's social and emotional development and improvement on responding appropriately to children who are distressed. Comments of the supervisors indicate that students improved in their ability to support challenging behaviors in the classroom, connect with parents and families, and provide children with positive and sensitive care: "She (student) really tuned into the children and their needs and has such a gentle and caring demeanor with them".

Other evidence of positive changes in the students is provided by their self-report of their confidence in demonstrating competencies needed to promote social and emotional development and to address challenging behaviors in young children (National Center on the Social and Emotional Foundations for Early Learning—CSEFEL). Results examining self-efficacy scores suggest students' knowledge and confidence improved in developing nurturing and responsive relationships, creating high quality environments, providing targeted social emotional supports, and implementing intensive interventions. That is, at the end of the program, students perceived themselves as more capable in competencies such as developing meaningful relationships with children and their families, structuring routines and providing environments that help young children learn, feel competent, and socialize with peers and adults, partnering and working with families from diverse backgrounds, and implementing assessments, observations, and intensive intervention activities.

In addition to providing support that the EC-SEBRIS program was successful in promoting positive outcomes for the ECE professionals (students) enrolled in the program, this study provides evidence that the program helped the children and families that the ECE professionals (students) served. Similarly, numerous studies on positive behavior support in ECE settings indicate that effective behavior management in the classrooms support young children's abilities to regulate their emotions and behaviors and yield better child outcomes [47–50]. The Parent surveys assessing their children's social competencies and behavioral challenges described by Desired Results Developmental Profile (DRDP) standards show that parents perceived positive social emotional gains for their children. Analyses revealed that parents recognized the improvement in their child's social competencies and behaviors, as they indicated that their child is able to regulate their emotions and behaviors, stopped biting, have less tantrums, and is able to use social skills to befriend the children around them. In open-ended comments, parents indicated the change in their child's social skills in the wake of the intervention. Parents wrote that their child is able to share, identify, and express emotions, problem-solve, manage strong emotions, and communicate needs. For example, according to one parent: "My child is literally a different person! She has become less violent and more compassionate towards other people. Prior to this program, my daughter had no friends. Now, she has friends and the kids actually want to play with her". Hence, positive sensitive teacher–child relationships appear to decrease behavioral challenges and the negative effects for children at risk for externalizing and internalizing problems [38,46].

The results presented on the EC-SEBRIS certificate program show that intensive training that combines knowledge, experience, and reflective practice support the professional growth in early childhood professionals and their ability to provide nurturing, sensitive, and responsive care to children. Analyses of behavioral observations of the ECE professionals (students) interacting with young children and site supervisors' report of the ECE professionals' competencies offer evidence that the program had positive effects on the ECE professionals' abilities to support young children's socio-emotional and behavior regulation. ECE professionals also gained a sense of self efficacy in their ability to understand behaviors and provide children with the appropriate support and regulation plan. In addition, the results suggest that the positive effects extended to the children served by the ECE professionals in the EC-SEBRIS program. That is, analyses of parent reports of their children's behaviors, as well as their open-ended comments, provide evidence that the children served by the ECE professionals made positive gains over the one-year EC-SEBRIS program.

Future research is needed to further examine the effects of the EC-SEBRIS program on the children served. Assessments that measure children's behaviors with targeted periodic observations in the classroom as well as at home are needed to confirm the current findings that were based solely on parent report. In addition, most of the participants in the EC-SEBRIS program, as well as in the field of early childhood education in general, are female. Future research should examine the generalizability of the current results and include a larger sample so that we can understand the characteristics of participants (e.g., gender, years of work in early childhood education, experience with mental health professionals) and children served (e.g., gender, age), which may influence the effectiveness of the

EC-SEBRIS program. Additionally, future studies should include a control group, and the long-term effects of the training on the ECE professionals and the children they served should be examined.

5. Conclusions

The EC-SEBRIS program presented above was designed to prepare a workforce of early childhood professionals to provide sensitive relational care and to address early mental health problems with behavior and emotional regulation. The one-year graduate certificate training program includes core content coursework, practicum experiences, and reflective supervision that was provided in individual and group sessions by an experienced licensed mental health professional. The use of videotaping for supervisors to provide instruction and encourage reflection, as well as on-site coaching at their practicum sites, were components facilitating the integration of theory to practice and skill building in the ECE professionals.

The EC-SEBRIS wraparound training and coaching model views the early childhood teacher/care educator as an important member of the first-response team to the child's needs and daily care. The EC-SEBRIS training equipped the teacher with the knowledge and skills to recognize the child's needs and come up with a response, which meets the child's needs. It is built on strength-based framework [81] in which teachers are trained to identify social competencies and capitalize on the strengths of children with challenging behaviors early on, rather than focusing on their problem behaviors. The program also recognizes that the stress, burnout, and frustration early childhood educators feel in their jobs affect their relationships with the children in their care and the environments they create for the children [51,52]. Thus, the program enhances ECE professionals' capacity to provide warm, responsive caregiving and reduce problem behaviors and rates of expulsion by giving them greater access to mental health consultation [5,53–55], as well as giving them direct training to increase their knowledge, skills, and competencies to support emotion and behavior regulation in young children under their care. The program equips the ECE professionals who work with young children on a daily basis with the skills and competencies to support children's healthy development, to address problem behaviors on-site, and to provide children with a safe, familiar adult who is able to "contain" their frustrations and temperaments. It also provides other teachers on-site with an opportunity to learn from their peers and model their behaviors and problem-solving practices. This study renders support to the assertion that professional training that focuses on emotional and behavior regulation support is essential for early childhood professionals working with young children [68].

Acknowledgments: The EC-SEBRIS Certificate Program has received funding from San Diego County Health and Human Services Administration (HHSA) Behavioral Health.

Author Contributions: Shulamit N. Ritblatt developed and implemented the EC-SEBRIS teaching model and the multi-years evaluation. She wrote the manuscript together with Audrey Hokoda who supported the evaluation process. Charles Van Liew is a consultant and provides support with data analyses. He provided this support to the program evaluation throughout the years. He ran the analyses and contributed to the writing of the methods and results. All authors reviewed the manuscript and provided final comments and suggestions.

Conflicts of Interest: The founding sponsors had no role in the design of the study; in the collection, analyses, or interpretation of data; in the writing of the manuscript; or in the decision to publish the results.

References

1. Lynda, L. *Who's Minding the Kids? Child. Care Arrangements: Spring 2011*; United States Census Bureau: Suitland, MD, USA, 2013.
2. Zero to Three. Infants and Toddlers and the California Mental Health Services Act. 2007. Available online: http://ceo.lacounty.gov/ccp/pdf/mhsa_pei/03InfantsandToddlersandMHSA.pdf (accessed on 20 June 2010).
3. Strain, P.S.; Joseph, G.E. Engaged supervision to support recommended practices for young children with challenging behavior. *Top. Early Child. Spec. Educ.* **2004**, *24*, 39–50. [CrossRef]
4. Gilliam, W.S. *Prekindergarteners Left Behind: Expulsion Rates in State Kindergarten Programs*; Foundation for Child Development (FCD): New York, NY, USA, 2005.

5. Gilliam, W. *Reducing Behavior Problems in Early Care and Education Programs: An Evaluation of Connecticut's Early Childhood Consultation Partnership*; Child Health and Development Institute of Connecticut, Inc.: Farmington, CT, USA, 2007.
6. Costello, E.J.; Maughan, B. Annual research review: Optimal outcomes of child and adolescent mental illness. *J. Child Psychol. Psychiatry* **2015**, *56*, 324–341. [CrossRef] [PubMed]
7. Jones, P.B. Adult mental health disorders and their age at onset. *Br. J. Psychiatry* **2013**, *202*, s5–s10. [CrossRef] [PubMed]
8. Van Der Ende, J.; Verhulst, C.F.; Tiemeier, H. The bidirectional pathways between internalizing and externalizing problems and academic performance from 6 to 18 years. *Dev. Psychopathol.* **2016**, *28*, 855–867. [CrossRef] [PubMed]
9. Cicchetti, D.; Toth, S.L. Child maltreatment. *Ann. Rev. Clin. Psychol.* **2005**, *1*, 409–438. [CrossRef] [PubMed]
10. DeWall, C.N.; Baumeister, R.F.; Stillman, T.F.; Gailliot, M.T. Violence restrained: Effects of self-regulation and its depletion on aggression. *J. Exp. Soc. Psychol.* **2007**, *43*, 62–76. [CrossRef]
11. Eisenberg, N.; Spinrad, T.L.; Eggum, N.D. Emotion-related self-regulation and its relation to children's maladjustment. *Ann. Rev. Clin. Psychol.* **2010**, *6*, 495–525. [CrossRef] [PubMed]
12. Quinn, P.D.; Fromme, K. Self-regulation as a protective factor against risky drinking and sexual behavior. *Psychol. Addict. Behav.* **2010**, *24*, 376–385. [CrossRef] [PubMed]
13. Anzman-Frasca, S.; Stifter, C.A.; Birch, L.L. Temperament and childhood obesity risk: A review of the literature. *J. Dev. Behav. Pediatr.* **2012**, *33*, 732–745. [CrossRef] [PubMed]
14. Graziano, P.A.; Calkins, S.D.; Keane, S.P. Toddler self-regulation skills predict risk for pediatric obesity. *Int. J. Obes.* **2010**, *34*, 633–641. [CrossRef] [PubMed]
15. Schwebel, D.C. Temperamental risk factors for children's unintentional injury: The role of impulsivity and inhibitory control. *Personal. Individ. Differ.* **2004**, *37*, 567–578. [CrossRef]
16. Center for Evidence-Based Practices: Young Children with Challenging Behavior. *Prevention and Intervention with Young Children's Challenging Behavior: A Consensus Based Summary of Current Knowledge*; University of South Florida: Tampa, FL, USA, 2005.
17. Blaze, J.; Roth, T.L. Caregiver maltreatment causes altered neuronal DNA methylation in female rodents. *Dev. Psychopathol.* **2017**, *29*, 477–489. [CrossRef] [PubMed]
18. Turp, M. Why love matters: How affection shapes a baby's brain: A review. *Infant Obs.* **2006**, *9*, 305–309.
19. Siegel, D.J.; Hartzell, M. *Parenting from the Inside Out*; Jeremy, P., Ed.; Tarcher/Penguin: New York, NY, USA, 2003.
20. Anda, R.F.; Felitti, V.; Bremer, D.; Walker, J.; Whitfield, C.; Perry, B.; Dube, S.; Giles, W. The enduring effects of abuse and related adverse experiences in childhood. A convergence of evidence from neurobiology and epidemiology. *Eur. Arch. Psychiatry Clin. Neurosci.* **2006**, *256*, 174–186. [CrossRef] [PubMed]
21. Fisher, H.; Cohen-Woods, S.; Hosang, G.M.; Korszun, A.; Owen, M.; Craddock, N.; Craig, I.W.; Farmer, A.E.; McGuffin, P.; Uher, R. Interaction between specific forms of childhood maltreatment and the serotonin transporter gene (*5-HTT*) in recurrent depressive disorder. *J. Affect. Disord.* **2013**, *145*, 136–141. [CrossRef] [PubMed]
22. Shonkoff, J.; Fisher, P. Rethinking evidence-based practice and two-generation programs to create the future of early childhood policy. *Dev. Psychopathol.* **2013**, *25*, 1635–1653. [CrossRef] [PubMed]
23. Meltzoff, A. Roots of social cognition: The like-me framework. In *Minnesota Symposia on Child Psychology: Meeting the Challenge of Translational Research in Child Psychology*; Cicchetti, D., Gunnar, M.R., Eds.; John Wiley: Hoboken, NJ, USA, 2009; pp. 29–55.
24. Dalli, C.; White, E.J.; Rockel, J.; Duhn, I.; Buchanan, E.; Davidson, S.; Ganly, S.; Kus, L.; Wang, B. *Quality Early Childhood Education for Under-Two-Year-Olds: What Should It Look Like? A literature Review*; Report to the Ministry of Education; New Zealand Ministry of Education: Wellington, New Zealand, 2011.
25. Herrod, H.G. Do first years really last a lifetime? *Clin. Pediatr.* **2007**, *46*, 199–205. [CrossRef] [PubMed]
26. Shonkoff, J.P. Building a new biodevelopmental framework to guide the future of early childhood policy. *Child Dev.* **2010**, *81*, 357–367. [CrossRef] [PubMed]
27. Center on the Developing Child at Harvard University. *The Foundations of Lifelong Health Are Built in Early Childhood*; Center on the Developing Child at Harvard University: Cambridge, MA, USA, 2010.
28. National Scientific Council on the Developing Child Harvard University. *Young Children Develop in an Environment of Relationships: Working Paper #1*; Harvard University: Cambridge, MA, USA, 2004.

29. National Scientific Council on the Developing Child. *Children's Emotional Development is Built into the Architecture of Their Brains: Working Paper #2*; Harvard University: Cambridge, MA, USA, 2004.

30. National Scientific Council on the Developing Child. *Excessive Stress Disrupts the Architecture of the Developing Brain: Working Paper #3*; Harvard University: Cambridge, MA, USA, 2005.

31. National Scientific Council on the Developing Child. *The Science of Early Childhood Development: Closing the Gap between what We Do and What We Know*; Harvard University: Cambridge, MA, USA, 2007.

32. Roisman, G.I.; Barnett-Walker, K.; Owen, M.T.; Bradley, R.H.; Steinberg, L.; Susman, E.; Booth-LaForce, C.; Belsky, J.; Houts, R. Early family and child-care antecedents of awakening cortisol levels in adolescence. *Child Dev.* **2009**, *80*, 907–920. [CrossRef] [PubMed]

33. Watamura, S.; Donzella, B.; Alwin, J.; Gunnar, M.R. Morning-to-afternoon increases in cortisol concentrations for infants and toddlers at child care age differences and behavioral correlates. *Child Dev.* **2003**, *74*, 1006–1020. [CrossRef] [PubMed]

34. Gerhardt, S. *Why Love Matters: How Affection Shapes a Baby's Brain*; Routledge: London, UK, 2004.

35. Gunnar, M.R.; Donzella, B. Social regulation of the cortisol levels in early human development. *Psychoneuroendocrinology* **2002**, *27*, 199–220. [CrossRef]

36. Sabol, T.; Pianta, R.C. Recent trends in research on teacher-child relationships. *Attach. Hum. Dev.* **2012**, *14*, 213–231. [CrossRef] [PubMed]

37. Buyse, E.; Verschueren, K.; Verachtert, P.; Van Damme, J. Predicting school adjustment in early elementary school: Impact of teacher-child relationship quality and relational classroom climate. *Elem. Sch. J.* **2009**, *110*, 119–141. [CrossRef]

38. Baker, J.A.; Grant, S.; Morlock, L. The teacher-student relationship as a developmental context for children with internalizing or externalizing behavior problems. *Sch. Psychol. Q.* **2008**, *23*, 3–15. [CrossRef]

39. Birch, S.H.; Ladd, G.W. The teacher-child relationship and children's early school adjustment. *J. Sch. Psychol.* **1997**, *35*, 61–79. [CrossRef]

40. Colwell, M.J.; Lindsey, E.W. *Preschool Children's Conflict and Social Competence: A Comparative View*; Undergraduate Research Community: Okemos, MI, USA, 2000.

41. Howes, C. 2000 Social-emotional classroom climate in child care, child-teacher relationships and children's second grade peer relations. *Soc. Dev.* **2000**, *9*, 191–204. [CrossRef]

42. Ladd, G.W.; Birch, S.H.; Buhs, E.S. Children's social and scholastic lives in kindergarten: Related spheres of influence. *Child Dev.* **1999**, *70*, 1373–1400. [CrossRef] [PubMed]

43. Lisonbee, J.A.; Mize, J.; Payne, A.L.; Granger, D.A. Children's cortisol and the quality of teacher-child relationships in child care. *Child Dev.* **2008**, *79*, 1818–1832. [CrossRef] [PubMed]

44. Palermo, F.; Hanish, L.D.; Martin, C.L.; Fabes, R.A.; Reiser, M. Preschoolers' academic readiness: What role does the teacher-child relationship play? *Early Child. Res. Q.* **2007**, *22*, 407–422. [CrossRef] [PubMed]

45. Pianta, R.C.; Stuhlman, M.W. Teacher-child relationships and children's success in the first years of school. *Sch. Psychol. Rev.* **2004**, *33*, 444–458.

46. Ladd, G.W.; Burgess, K.B. Do relational risks and protective factors moderate the linkages between childhood aggression and early psychological and school adjustment? *Child Dev.* **2001**, *72*, 1579–1601. [CrossRef] [PubMed]

47. Conners-Burrow, N.A.; Whiteside-Mansell, L.; Mckelvey, L.; Virmani, E.A.; Sockwell, L. Improved classroom quality and child behavior in an Arkansas early childhood mental health consultation pilot project. *Infant Ment. Health J.* **2012**, *33*, 256–264. [CrossRef] [PubMed]

48. Fabiano, G.A.; Vujnovic, R.K.; Waschbusch, D.A.; Yu, J.; Mashtare, T.; Pariseau, M.E.; Pelham, W.E.; Parhama, B.R.; Smalls, K.J. Comparison of workshop training versus intensive, experiential training for improving behavior support skills in early educators. *Early Child. Res. Q.* **2013**, *28*, 450–460. [CrossRef]

49. Landry, S.H.; Anthony, J.L.; Swank, P.R.; Pauline Monseque-Bailey, P. Effectiveness of comprehensive professional development for teachers of at-risk preschoolers. *J. Educ. Psychol.* **2009**, *101*, 448–465. [CrossRef]

50. Raver, C.C.; Jones, S.M.; Li-Grining, C.; Zhai, F.; Metzger, M.W.; Solomon, B. Targeting children's behavior problems in preschool classrooms: A cluster-randomized controlled trial. *J. Consult. Clin. Psychol.* **2009**, *77*, 302–316. [CrossRef] [PubMed]

51. Lambert, R.G.; McCarthy, C.J.; O'Donnell, M.; Wang, C. Measuring elementary teacher stress and coping in the classroom: Validity evidence for the classroom appraisal of resources and demands. *Psychol. Sch.* **2009**, *46*, 973–988. [CrossRef]

52. Li-Grining, C.P.; Votruba-Drzal, E.; Maldonado-Carreño, C.; Haas, K. Children's early approaches to learning and academic trajectories through fifth grade. *Dev. Psychol.* **2010**, *46*, 1062. [CrossRef] [PubMed]

53. Brennan, M. "They Just Want to be with Us": Young Children Learning to Live the Culture: A Post-Vygotskian Analysis of Young Children's Enculturation into a Childcare Setting. Ph.D. Thesis, Victoria University of Wellington, Wellington, New Zealand, 2005.

54. Perry, D.; Dunne, M.C.; McFadden, L.; Campbell, D. Reducing the risk for preschool expulsion: Mental health consultation for young children with challenging behaviors. *J. Child Family Stud.* **2008**, *17*, 44–54. [CrossRef]

55. Upshur, C.; Wenz-Gross, M.; Reed, G. A pilot study of early childhood mental health consultation for children with behavioral problems in preschool. *Early Child. Res. Q.* **2009**, *24*, 29–45. [CrossRef]

56. Gilliam, W.; Shahar, G. Preschool and child care expulsion and suspension: Rates and predictors in one state. *Infants Young Child.* **2006**, *19*, 228–245. [CrossRef]

57. Alkon, A.; Ramler, M.; MacLennan, K. Evaluation of mental health consultation in child care centers. *Early Child. Educ. J.* **2003**, *31*, 91–99. [CrossRef]

58. Brennan, E.M.; Bradley, J.R.; Allan, D.M.; Perry, D.F. The evidence base for mental health consultation in early childhood settings: Research synthesis addressing staff and program outcomes. *J. Early Educ. Dev.* **2008**, *19*, 982–1022. [CrossRef]

59. Conners-Burrow, N.A.; Kramer, T.L.; Sigel, B.A.; Helpenstill, K.; Sievers, C.; McKelvey, L. Trauma-informed care training in a child welfare system: Moving it to the front line. *Child. Youth Serv. Rev.* **2013**, *35*, 1830–1835. [CrossRef]

60. Green, B.; Simpson, J.; Everhart, M.; Vale, E.; Gettman, M. Understanding integrated mental health services in Head Start: Staff perspectives on mental health consultation. *Natl. Head Start Assoc. Dialogue* **2004**, *7*, 35–60. [CrossRef]

61. Green, B.L.; Everhart, M.; Gordon, L.; Gettman, M.G. Characteristics of effective mental health consultation in early childhood settings: Multilevel analysis of a national survey. *Top. Early Child. Spec. Educ.* **2006**, *26*, 142–152. [CrossRef]

62. Virmani, E.A.; Masyn, K.E.; Thompson, R.A.; Conners-Burrow, N.; Whiteside-Mansell, L. Early childhood mental health consultation: Promoting change in quality of teacher-child interactions. *Infant Ment. Health J.* **2013**, *34*, 156–172. [CrossRef]

63. Virmani, E.; Ontai, L.L. Supervision and training in child care: Does reflective supervision foster caregiver insightfulness? *Infant Ment. Health J.* **2010**, *31*, 16–32. [CrossRef] [PubMed]

64. Fonagy, P.; Target, M.; Steele, H.; Steele, M. *Reflective-Functioning Manual Version 5 for Application to Adult Attachment Interviews*; University College London: London, UK, 1998.

65. Gatti, S.N.; Watson, C.L.; Siegel, C.F. Step back and consider: Learning from reflective practice in infant mental health. *Young Except. Child.* **2011**, *14*, 32–45. [CrossRef]

66. Koren-Karie, N.; Oppenheim, D.; Dolve, S.; Sher, E.; Etzion-Carasso, E. Mother's insightfulness regarding their infant's internal experience: Relations with maternal sensitivity and infant attachment. *Dev. Psychol.* **2002**, *38*, 534–542. [CrossRef] [PubMed]

67. Slade, A.; Grienenberger, J.; Bernbach, E.; Levy, D.; Locker, A. Maternal reflective functioning and attachment: Considering the transmission gap. *Attach. Hum. Dev.* **2005**, *7*, 283–296. [CrossRef] [PubMed]

68. Fox, L.; Dunlap, G.; Hemmeter, M.L.; Joseph, G.; Strain, P. The teaching pyramid: Model for supporting social competence and preventing challenging behavior in young children. *Young Child.* **2003**, *58*, 48–53.

69. Ritblatt, S.N. Early Childhood Socio-Emotional and Behavior Regulation Intervention Specialist (EC-SEBRIS) training model: A crossroad of mental health and early childhood education. *J. Ment. Health Train. Educ. Pract.* **2016**, *11*, 1–13. [CrossRef]

70. Huhra, R.L. Reviewing videotape in supervision: A developmental approach. *J. Couns. Dev.* **2008**, *86*, 412–418. [CrossRef]

71. Romans, J.C.; Boswell, D.L.; Carlozzi, A.F.; Ferguson, D.B. Training and supervision practices in clinical, counseling, and school psychology programs. *Prof. Psychol. Res. Pract.* **1995**, *26*, 407–412. [CrossRef]

72. Zan, B.; Donegan-Ritter, M. Reflecting, coaching and mentoring to enhance teacher–child interactions in Head Start classroom. *Early Child. Educ. J.* **2014**, *42*, 93–104. [CrossRef]

73. California Infant, Preschool & Family Mental Health Initiative. *The Delivery of Infant Family and Early Mental Health Services: Training Guidelines and Recommended Personnel Competencies*; WestEd Center for Prevention and Early Intervention: Sacramento, CA, USA, 2010.

74. Pianta, R.C.; Mashburn, A.J.; Downer, J.T.; Hamre, B.K.; Justice, L. Effects of web-mediated professional development resources on teacher-child interactions in pre-kindergarten classrooms. *Early Child. Res. Q.* **2008**, *23*, 431–451. [CrossRef] [PubMed]

75. Blair, K.S.C.; Fox, L.; Lentini, R. Use of positive behavior support to address the challenging behavior of young children within a community early childhood program. *Top. Early Child. Spec. Educ.* **2010**, *30*, 68–79. [CrossRef]

76. Joyce, B.R.; Showers, B. *Student Achievement through Staff Development*, 3rd ed.; Association for Supervision & Curriculum Development (ASCD): Alexandria, VA, USA, 2002.

77. Tout, K.; Isner, T.; Zaslow, M. Coaching for Quality Improvement: Lessons Learned from Quality Rating and Improvement Systems. In *Research brief for the Children's Services Council of Palm Beach County*; Child Trends: Washington, DC, USA, 2011.

78. Arnett, J. Caregivers in day-care centers: Does training matter? *J. Appl. Dev. Psychol.* **1989**, *10*, 541–552. [CrossRef]

79. Colwell, N.; Gordon, R.A.; Ken Fujimoto, K.; Robert Kaestner, R.; Korenmane, S. New evidence on the validity of the Arnett Caregiver Interaction Scale: Results from the Early Childhood Longitudinal Study-Birth Cohort. *Early Child. Res. Q.* **2013**, *28*, 218–233. [CrossRef] [PubMed]

80. Campbell, P.H.; Milbourne, S.A. Improving the quality of infant—Toddler care through professional development. *Top. Early Child. Spec. Educ.* **2005**, *25*, 3–14. [CrossRef]

81. Sutherland, K.S.; Conroy, M.A.; Abrams, L.; Vo, A. Improving interactions between teachers and young children with problem behavior: A strengths-based approach. *Exceptionality* **2010**, *18*, 70–81. [CrossRef]

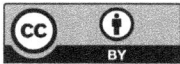

Article

Child Community Mental Health Services in Asia Pacific and Singapore's REACH Model

Choon Guan Lim *, Hannah Loh, Vidhya Renjan, Jason Tan and Daniel Fung

Department of Child and Adolescent Psychiatry, Institute of Mental Health, Singapore 539747, Singapore;
hannah_yl_loh@imh.com.sg (H.L.); vidhya_renjan@imh.com.sg (V.R.); Jason_ZX_TAN@imh.com.sg (J.T.);
Daniel_Fung@imh.com.sg (D.F.)
* Correspondence: choon_guan_lim@imh.com.sg; Tel.: +65-6389-2000

Received: 31 July 2017; Accepted: 27 September 2017; Published: 6 October 2017

Abstract: In recent decades, there have been concerted efforts to improve mental health services for youths alongside the challenges of rising healthcare costs and increasing demand for mental health needs. One important phenomenon is the shift from traditional clinic-based care to community-based mental health services to improve accessibility to services and provide patient-centred care. In this article, we discuss the child and adolescent community mental health efforts within the Asia-Pacific region. We also discuss Singapore's community and school-based mental health service, known as the Response, Early Intervention and Assessment in Community Mental Health (REACH). This article discusses how REACH has evolved over the years in response to the changing needs of youths in Singapore. Finally, we discuss the current challenges and future directions for youth mental health care.

Keywords: child psychiatry; community mental health; school-based mental health; mental health service

1. Burden of Mental Health in Young People

1.1. Overview

It is reported that 1 in 10 children experience mental health problems but less than a third of them are likely to seek help [1]. Furthermore, mental health disorders in youths are often not detected till much later in life [2]. Globally, mental disorders account for a significant portion of disease burden in youths, with poor mental health impacting the young person's physical health and development by affecting their academic and vocational achievements, social relationships, and exposing them to stigma and discrimination [1–3]. Poor youth mental health is also significantly associated with maladaptive substance use, violence and increased mortality rates due to suicide, self-harm, and accidental harm which further increases health-care costs [1,2].

1.2. Greater Push towards Improving Mental Health Support for Children and Adolescents

Historically, a larger proportion of mental health services and resources have been channeled towards treating older and chronic populations. Treating youths required specialized child-friendly and youth-oriented therapeutic approaches with few psychiatrists and professionals choosing to specialize in this area, particularly in the Asia-Pacific region. Diagnosing youths can be challenging due to multiple psycho-social influences, and often requires a multi-disciplinary, inter-agency approach to treatment and care [2].

However, over the past four decades, efforts to improve the mental health treatment and services for children and adolescents have grown considerably [4]. Increasingly, governments and global healthcare organizations, such as the World Health Organization (WHO), recognize the burden of mental disorders in youths and have moved towards prevention, earlier identification and intervention, and improving mental health resilience amongst youths [5,6]. For example, in 2005 the WHO promulgated its Mental Health Policy and Service Guidance Package to provide specific guidelines to healthcare makers and governments on policy development and service delivery of child and adolescent mental health services [7].

1.3. Singapore

Singapore is a small island-state located within Southeast Asia. Its population is multi-ethnic, with Chinese making the majority at 74%, followed by Malays (13%), Indians (9%), and other ethnic minorities (3%). As of 2016, Singapore had approximately 835,900 children and adolescents below the age of 20 years [8]. In the only community-based prevalence study involving 2139 school-going children aged 6 to 12 years, the prevalence of emotional and behavioral problems was found to be comparable to studies in the West at 12.5% [9]. The same study also found the prevalence of internalizing disorders to be more than twice that of externalizing disorders which was in contrast to studies in the West. In a 2010 study on disease burden amongst Singapore residents, mental disorders accounted for the largest portion, about one-third of disability-adjusted life years (DALYs), in children aged below 15 years. Specifically, autism spectrum disorder, attention-deficit/hyperactivity disorder, and anxiety and depression were amongst the top 10 causes of disability burden amongst children between the ages of 0 and 14 years. Amongst young people between the ages of 15 and 34 years, mental disorders—mainly schizophrenia, and anxiety and depression—accounted for a significantly greater burden, approximately 19% DALYs, within this age group [10]. Suicide rate is one of the surrogate indicators to measure mental well-being of a society. Among young people in Singapore, the suicide rate was 5.7 per 100,000 and closely associated with psychosocial stressors, including academic stress [11,12]. An analysis of global suicide rates in 81 countries, between 1990 and 2009, showed a declining trend in average suicide rates of youths aged between 15 and 19 years. Globally, the average suicide rate for males decreased from 10.32 to 9.50 (per 100,000) and the suicide rate for females remained steady at 4.41 to 4.19 (per 100,000). In Europe, the average suicide rate showed a significant decline for both genders, decreasing from 13.13 to 10.93 (per 100,000) in males and from 3.88 to 3.34 (per 100,000) in females. In the United States, there was a significant decrease in suicide rates for males (16.13 to 11.81 per 100,000) and females (3.31 to 2.82 per 100,000). In Australia, there was a significant decline in suicides for males 15 to 19 years (16.79 to 11.10 per 100,000), while rates remained stable for females (4.12 to 4.17 per 100,000). However, the authors note that limited data exists for African and Asian countries, and further examination of suicide rates in these regions is required to aid in cross-cultural comparisons [13].

Demand for services at the outpatient child and adolescent psychiatric clinic (Child Guidance Clinic, or CGC) of the Institute of Mental Health (IMH), Singapore's only tertiary-care psychiatric hospital, has steadily increased over the years. The number of new cases seen has risen six-fold from approximately 500 new cases annually in the 1980s to almost 3000 annually by 2010 [14]. This increase is concerning and while it may be due to the clinic's outreach effort to the schools and greater awareness of mental disorders in the community rather than an actual increase in the incidence of mental disorders, it exerts a strain on the clinic's resources. Additionally, to improve clinical outcome, there is a need to focus on prevention and providing care further upstream. The current clinic-based model does not seem ideal to fulfill these roles.

2. Global Trends in Community Mental Health Efforts

Past models of care depended on mental health professionals for direct service delivery. However, the shortage of trained mental healthcare professionals make provision of future direct services in outpatient and inpatient settings unsustainable due to rapid growing demands and costs. There is also pressure on mental health services to provide appropriate and timely services that are sustainable and cost-effective [15]. With the push to deinstitutionalize mental healthcare and move towards a tiered approach in mental healthcare provision, there is a shift towards establishing community-based mental health services [16].

The WHO's Comprehensive Mental Health Action Plan 2013–2020, for example, calls for member states to "provide comprehensive, integrated and responsive mental health and social care services in community-based settings" to improve access of care and service quality [17]. Other benefits of community-based care include early access to intervention, increased treatment adherence, human rights protection, prevention of stigma, reduced hospital admissions, and fewer deaths by suicide [18].

3. Child and Adolescent Community Mental Health Efforts across the Asia-Pacific Region

Community mental healthcare is still in a nascent stage of development in the Asia-Pacific region, with governments and service providers working collaboratively together only in the last decade to increase funding, and establish policies and guidelines on community mental healthcare. Such developments include the establishment of the Asia-Pacific Community Mental Health Development (APCMHD) project in 2005 by 14 member nations to promote information exchange on best practices within the region [19].

3.1. Increased Accessibility to Community Mental Health Teams and Centers

A key feature of many community mental health models is the establishment of mental health teams and centers within the community to increase accessibility of services. Community mental health teams are usually multi-disciplinary in nature comprising psychiatrists, psychologists, occupational therapists, social workers, nurses, and other allied health professionals, who are situated in community mental health centers located conveniently in districts and bureaus across the country.

For instance, in Hong Kong, the Social Welfare Department introduced the Integrated Community Center for Mental Wellness (ICCMW) initiative in 2010, a one-stop, integrated, district-based center where people with mental health problems can access mental health services at designated centers across different districts [20].

Increasingly, community mental health teams have focused specifically on servicing children and adolescents. As of 2004, 24 community mental health centers in South Korea engaged in school mental health services to neighboring schools [21]. In Taiwan and Singapore, specialized early intervention centers have been established since the mid-2000s to provide assessment and intervention services to children with developmental delays and their families [22].

3.2. Increased Patient-Centered Innovation

A shift towards community care also signals a shift in attitude towards organizing care around patients' needs. Increasingly, governments and healthcare providers are designing services that are integrated, comprehensive, flexible, and responsive to overcome challenges that patients encounter in accessing mental health services, including stigma, proximity to services, and lack of continuity of care. In Taiwan for example, the "Taipei Model" developed by the Taipei City Psychiatric Center (TCPC) seeks to integrate community mental healthcare services within the primary care and general healthcare system. Under this model, public health workers from 12 district health centers provide follow-up visits to patients who were recently discharged from the TCPC to ensure that there is continuity of care to patients [19].

To make mental healthcare services accessible to youths living in rural parts of Australia, the "headspace" program was established in 2006 to minimize stigma and aid in the promotion and early intervention of mental health problems for youth aged 12 to 25 years [23]. Additionally, "headspace" was designed to integrate mental and physical health services to provide a one-stop stigma-free service for youths who often presented with a comorbid of physical and mental health problems. In an evaluation study of "headspace", both clinicians and youths reported that the co-location of medical and counselling services within the service encouraged help-seeking behavior, while youths reported increased likelihood of treatment adherence [24].

Moreover, mental healthcare providers in Australia have innovated services to meet the needs of the population. For instance, "ReachOut", established in 1998, is Australia's leading online mental health service for youths which aims to provide youths with easy access to 24/7 anonymous help by employing online technology [25].

3.3. Increased Government Funding and Support

Across Asia, governments have also increased funding earmarked for community mental health efforts, and pushed for a more comprehensive system of care. Recently in Singapore, an additional funding of S$160 million has been ring-fenced to increase community mental health services as part of a five-year Community Mental Health Masterplan from 2017 to 2021. Governments in the region have also pushed for preventative care and early intervention as part of community-based mental healthcare, targeting children and adolescents. For example, the South Korean 2005 Mental Health Services guidelines recognizes that critical aspects of child and adolescent mental health services include the prevention of mental health problems, early detection of such problems, and easier access to suitable treatments [21].

4. Singapore's Response

From a Singapore perspective, many mental disorders, including anxiety and depressive disorders, have onset in the childhood and adolescent years but remain untreated [26]. This emphasizes the need for early identification and intervention. Under the traditional model of care, a number of challenges with healthcare service delivery for youths were highlighted, such as long wait times, lack of appropriate and specialized care, fragmentation of service delivery within public health and social agencies, and duplication of services [27]. Stigma also notably plays a significant role for many Singaporean families, which may lead some to seek practitioners of traditional medicine or spiritual healers, consequently delaying access to appropriate and timely help [26,28]. Voluntary welfare organizations and initiatives, such as the Silver Ribbon Project and Singapore Association of Mental Health (SAMH), have been active in addressing stigma through public education, awareness programs and encouraging seeking early treatment. Furthermore, these programs portray individuals with mental health issues in a positive light and focus on building self-esteem and psychological health aspects. In addition, public education programs are also conducted in schools to promote mental health literacy. For youths between 16 and 30 years, the Community Health Assessment Team (CHAT), located at SCAPE Youth Park in the main city district, provides a one-stop center (CHAT Hub) for mental health assistance and resources [29].

In 2007, the National Mental Health Blueprint was developed to encourage primary prevention and monitoring of mental health of the population, improving service delivery and quality of psychiatric services, developing the mental health workforce, and promoting mental health research. Part of the vision under the 2007–2012 National Mental Health Blueprint included the right-siting and deinstitutionalization of care, leading to the inception of community-based services.

5. The REACH Model of Care

5.1. The Inception and Initial Years of REACH

In 2007, Response, Early Intervention and Assessment in Community Mental Health (REACH) was developed to support school-going students with mental health problems. Since 2003, compulsory education was enforced in Singapore and today, the compulsory school age is 6 to 15 years. The three main objectives of REACH are:

- improve mental health of youth via early assessment and intervention;
- build the capacity of schools and community partners to detect and manage mental health problems through support and training;
- build a community mental health support network for children and adolescents in the community, consisting of schools, general practitioners (GPs), and voluntary welfare organizations (VWOs).

The REACH model (see Figure 1) operates on regional hospital systems to create regional networks of mental healthcare and social services for seamless continuum of care for children and their families. The conception of REACH creates responsive services based on five criteria of quality care that is effective, accessible, timely, affordable, and safe as the central support mechanisms.

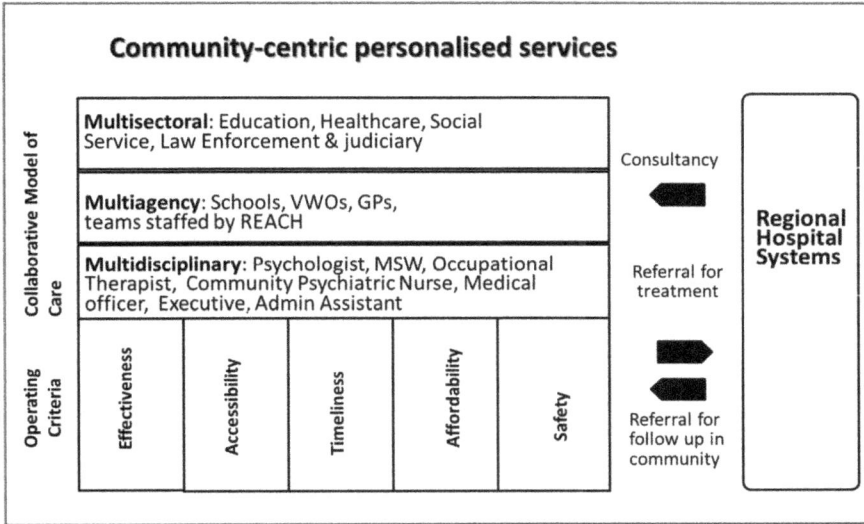

Figure 1. The REACH model of care. Note: VWOs = Voluntary Welfare Organizations; GPs = General Practitioners; MSW = Medical Social Worker.

REACH consists of four teams that service the north, south, east, and west geographical zones of Singapore, corresponding to the school zones [28]. Each team is comprised of a mobile multi-disciplinary team of medical doctors, psychologists, medical social workers, occupational therapists, and psychiatric nurses. REACH provides its services to schools primarily, and will provide assessment and appropriate intervention for students referred by the school counselor for mental health concerns. They also partner and engage VWOs (non-profit organizations that provide welfare services and/or services that aid the community) in providing services to these students and their families. By tapping on the provision of allied health services in schools, delivery of care via schools is envisioned to aid and increase mental wellness among school students. The REACH program is gradually phased to allow refinement of the program at each step.

The involvement of schools and community agencies reflects the global shift to a multi-sectoral and multi-agency tiered approach of care. Within school support services, teachers with basic counseling and behavioral management skills provide first-level intervention to students with socio-emotional and behavioral problems. At the next level, allied educators (mainstream schools) and allied health professionals (special schools) provide care to students who required specialized attention. For those who required intensive intervention or attention may be referred to specialists at the Ministry or external agencies such as hospital-based clinics or VWOs. Traditional clinic-based care for youths with mental health problems almost always involves collaborative care with schools and/or social agencies. Through the community-based care provided by REACH, the physical barrier in care coordination was bridged. Existing support networks further strengthened REACH teams to be mobile and provide assessment and intervention within schools or at home, thus, increasing accessibility of services and understanding of the child's problems within their naturalistic environment. Furthermore, the accessibility of REACH teams helps to reduce default rates of appointment, thereby increasing adherence to treatment and time to seek help [27].

The consultation helpline plays an integral role in REACH's service delivery. First, it increases timely accessibility to care. Secondly, cases that are referred via the helpline are tabled for discussion and triaged according to priority. School counsellors first gather relevant preliminary information regarding the child's mental health prior to contacting the REACH consultation helpline. However, there are limitations related to the varying clinical knowledge and understanding of school counsellors. Nevertheless, school counsellors and REACH teams work in collaboration to ensure that critical referral information is gathered. It should also be noted there is a designated REACH member assigned to each school who provides consultation to school counsellors when required. The referral is then tabled for discussion with the rest of the REACH multidisciplinary team to determine its appropriateness for referral for a more comprehensive mental health assessment. Cases that are deemed to have insufficient evidence for a mental health problem are provided recommendations for alternative support. This ensures an effective utilization of the team's resources. Apart from providing care, REACH also focuses on building the clinical capacity of school counsellors, VWOs, and community partners, by providing specialist training in early detection and management of common mental health problems seen among children and adolescents. Community partners of REACH are also invited to trainings by overseas mental health experts and monthly inter-agency case conferences to increase their clinical knowledge and aptitude in detection and management of mental health needs [27]. The engagement and collaboration of the network of agencies ensures that fragmentation of care and larger systemic issues are addressed. Table 1 shows the breakdown of diagnoses seen by REACH in 2015. Attention-Deficit Hyperactivity Disorder (ADHD) was the most commonly seen mental health disorder. Emotional disorders, including anxiety and mood disorders, were the second most commonly seen disorders by REACH teams.

Table 1. Breakdown by diagnosis for the cases seen in 2015.

Diagnosis	No. (%) of Cases
Attention-deficit hyperactivity disorder	247 (35.7)
Emotional disorder	159 (23.0)
No mental illness	133 (19.2)
Adjustment disorder	69 (10.0)
Developmental disorder	36 (5.2)
Conduct disorder	29 (4.2)
Others	18 (2.6)

Note: Emotional disorder includes anxiety and mood disorders; Adjustment disorder includes all stress-related disorders including situational reaction and adjustment disorder); Developmental disorder includes learning/developmental disorders and autism spectrum disorders; Conduct disorder includes cconduct disorder, oppositional defiant disorder, and mixed emotional and conduct disorder.

In a review of the effectiveness of the REACH program in terms of outcomes and effectiveness between 2007 and February 2015, 4184 students were referred to REACH by school counsellors. Out of these students, about 955 students were referred to tertiary specialist care. Clinical outcomes are measured by counsellor and teacher ratings on the Clinical Global Impression (CGI) scale [30] and Strength and Difficulties Questionnaire (SDQ; [31]), respectively. These measures are completed at intake assessment and six months post-assessment, regardless of whether the child receives intervention. These outcomes are presented in Table 2. In general, improvements in conduct problems, emotional problems, hyperactive behaviors and peer problems, and prosocial behavior on the SDQ and CGI severity of illness significantly improved after six months. Furthermore, findings show that community-based care compared to hospital-based care was more cost-effective, at a negative incremental cost-effectiveness ratio of S$18,308 per quality-adjusted life year (QALY) gained and maintained cost-effectiveness over the 95% confidence interval of QALY estimates [32,33].

Table 2. Means and standard deviations of clinical outcomes at pre and post (six-month) assessment.

	Pre-Assessment		Post Six-Month		
	Mean	**SD**	**Mean**	**SD**	*t*-test
CGI	3.14	0.11	2.42	0.06	17.88 **
SDQ-Emotional Problem	2.76	0.33	2.13	0.33	3.51 **
SDQ-Conduct	3.17	0.56	2.61	0.70	7.34 **
SDQ-Hyperactivity	6.71	0.46	6.01	0.41	12.18 **
SDQ-Peer problem	3.93	0.22	3.45	0.31	10.01 **
SDQ-Prosocial	4.05	0.30	4.47	0.70	−2.27 *

Note: CGI = Clinical Global Impression scale. SDQ = Strength & Difficulties Questionnaire. * $p = 0.05$, ** $p < 0.01$. Higher scores on the SDQ-prosocial behavior scale reflect desired behaviors.

Anecdotally, REACH services appear to be well-received by schools, as it is based in the community setting and is less stigmatizing in providing early assessment and intervention for youths. School leaders and counsellors have also given positive feedback on REACH teams' responsiveness to their schools' needs. In addition, schools have commended REACH team members' professional knowledge, communication skills, and provision of recommendations and care management plans to address the needs of each child. Conversely, for school staff who may not be aware of REACH services, REACH continues to generate awareness of its services through regular mental health literacy trainings to teachers in schools. Regular dialogues and reviews are also conducted inter-ministry, between REACH representatives (falling under the purview of the Ministry of Health) and the Ministry of Education (MOE), to address the changing needs of students and schools.

5.2. The Evolution of REACH

Since its inception, REACH has evolved to keep up with the changing needs and demands. There have been notable service developments to increase collaboration with community agencies and caregivers of the students seen by REACH. These included greater engagement with the MOE to streamline referral processes and improve inter-professional liaison and joint management of cases, partnership with specialized intervention centers to provide evidence-based intervention programs for children with co-morbid conditions such as dyslexia and conduct problems. Through collaboration, REACH also provides training workshops to equip school counselors and community partners with technical knowledge about specific mental illness, and intervention techniques such as motivational interviewing, mindfulness, and sensory-based strategies.

In 2016, REACH started a triage service for outpatient referrals made by regional polyclinics to CGC so as to arrange suitable cases for school-based assessment. Out of the 820 referrals from polyclinics, 279 (34%) were eventually assessed by REACH. Consequently, first visit wait-times were reduced at CGC. Re-directing appropriate referrals to REACH also aids in increasing catchment areas for responsive service provision.

6. Challenges and Future Considerations

On a global scale, major treatment gaps in addressing mental health problems exist, including a lack of manpower and clinical capacity of the mental healthcare workforce, varying political support of mental healthcare infrastructure and implementation of policies, and evaluation of novel and accessible models of care [34].

In Singapore, the REACH model of care has progressed to provide effective, timely, and accessible mental health service to children and adolescents. Despite the positive impact of the program, future directions include improving the processes in right-siting of referrals, continued capacity building of the REACH team and our stakeholders, and expansion of our collaboration with more school partners.

In addition to triaging outpatient referrals, REACH has also been looking to offer more group-based therapies to treat students presenting with mild mental health needs to more efficiently

Brain Sci. **2017**, 7, 126

meet the increased demand of services. Also, REACH is looking towards leveraging information technology systems to enhance all areas of service delivery. This includes using data analytic techniques to analyze trends in case referrals, and possibly tapping into technology-based assessment and therapy platforms. While initially conceptualized to provide services to children with mild mental health needs, the REACH program has now come to service children with more complex needs who prefer community care as opposed to secondary and tertiary psychiatric care. To meet the challenge of assessing and treating students with more complex difficulties, REACH team members would have to continually build competence through regular case discussions, supervision, and training. Besides having a background of providing cognitive-behavioral therapy, REACH psychologists are building competencies in third-wave therapies including mindfulness and acceptance and commitment therapy, whilst REACH occupational therapists build on sensory integration techniques, and occupational engagement. Given the larger systemic issues seen in children, REACH team members also receive training on evidence-based parenting programs such as the "Incredible Years" [35] and "Triple P" [36] programs. REACH also recognizes that fellow school and community partners have differing levels of competence which poses a challenge of catering to their varying training needs. Newer school and community partners may require more extensive training in basic mental health support strategies and require greater support from REACH teams.

As part of our commitment to reach out and make mental healthcare more accessible, future plans include expanding collaborations to a larger age-range by including preschools, and institutes of higher learning (e.g., polytechnics and universities). Concurrently, REACH continues to strengthen current partnerships with schools by promoting the development of whole-school approaches to support positive mental health and resilience in children by enhancing mental health literacy in the curriculum, and fostering a resilient culture that supports positive emotional well-being.

Another important aspect is the exchanging of our experience in providing school-based mental health care with our south-east Asian and Asian colleagues. While we may share some similar culture, educational, and health systems do vary from country to country. Over the years, we have shared our experiences in several regional conferences in China, Japan, Korea, Malaysia, and Indonesia. We will continue to maintain our professional networks so that we can continue to be updated on regional developments in youth mental health care services, especially in the context of community mental health services. For example, in the local residency program for child and adolescent psychiatry, overseas clinical fellowships are encouraged to enrich the experience of the next generation of psychiatrists.

Acknowledgments: We will like to acknowledge the help of all the schools which have been supported by the REACH teams.

Author Contributions: All the authors contributed substantially to the writing of the manuscript and are involved in the REACH program.

Conflicts of Interest: The authors declare no conflict of interest.

References

1. Kaushik, A.; Kostaki, E.; Kyriakopoulos, M. The stigma of mental illness in children and adolescents: A systematic review. *Psychiatry Res.* **2016**, *243*, 469–494. [CrossRef] [PubMed]
2. Patel, V.; Flisher, A.J.; Hetrick, S.; McGorry, P. Mental health of young people: A global public-health challenge. *Lancet* **2007**, *369*, 1302–1313. [CrossRef]
3. Whiteford, H.A.; Ferrari, A.J.; Degenhardt, L.; Feigin, V.; Vos, T. The global burden of mental, neurological and substance use disorders: An analysis from the global burden of disease study 2010. *PLoS ONE* **2015**, *10*, e0116820. [CrossRef] [PubMed]
4. Garland, A.F.; Haine-Schlagel, R.; Brookman-Frazee, L.; Baker-Ericzen, M.; Trask, E.; Fawley-King, K. Improving community-based mental health care for children: Translating knowledge into action. *Adm. Policy Ment. Health* **2013**, *40*, 6–22. [CrossRef] [PubMed]

5. Jorm, A.F. Mental health literacy: Empowering the community to take action for better mental health. *Am. Psychol.* **2012**, *67*, 231–243. [CrossRef] [PubMed]

6. Kelly, C.M.; Jorm, A.F.; Wright, A. Improving mental health literacy as a strategy to facilitate early intervention for mental disorders. *Med. J. Aust.* **2007**, *187*, S26–S30. [PubMed]

7. World Health Organization. Mental Health Policy and Service Guidance Package: Child and Adolescent Mental Health Policies and Plans. Available online: http://www.who.int/mental_health/policy/services/9_child%20ado_WEB_07.pdf (accessed on 21 June 2017).

8. Singapore Department of Statistics. Available online: http://www.singstat.gov.sg/statistics/latest-data#18 (accessed on 4 July 2017).

9. Woo, B.S.; Chang, W.C.; Fung, D.S.; Koh, J.B.; Leong, J.S.; Kee, C.H.; Seah, C.K. Development and validation of a depression scale for Asian adolescents. *J. Adolesc.* **2004**, *27*, 677–689. [CrossRef] [PubMed]

10. Ministry of Health Singapore. Singapore Burden of Disease Study 2010 Report. Available online: https://www.moh.gov.sg/content/dam/moh_web/Publications/Reports/2014/Singapore%20Burden%20of%20Disease%20Study%202010%20Report_v3.pdf (accessed on 19 June 2017).

11. Loh, C.; Tai, B.-C.; Ng, W.-Y.; Chia, A.; Chia, B.-H. Suicide in young Singaporeans aged 10–24 years between 2000 and 2004. *Arch. Suicide Res.* **2012**, *16*, 174–182. [CrossRef] [PubMed]

12. Ung, E.K. Youth suicide and parasuicide in Singapore. *Ann. Acad. Med. Singap.* **2003**, *32*, 12–18. [PubMed]

13. Kõlves, K.; De Leo, D. Adolescent suicide rates between 1990 and 2009: Analysis of age group 15–19 years worldwide. *J. Adolesc. Health* **2016**, *58*, 69–77. [CrossRef] [PubMed]

14. Tay, S.L.; Chan, M.C.; Fung, D. The vision. In *Reach Chronicles: A Community Mental Health Model for Children and Adolescents in Singapore*; Fung, D., Ong, L.P., Tay, S.L., Sim, W.H., Eds.; World Scientific: Singapore, 2012; pp. 19–72.

15. Hosie, A.; Vogl, G.; Hoddinott, J.; Carden, J.; Comeau, Y. Crossroads: Rethinking the Australian Mental Health System. Available online: http://about.au.reachout.com/wp-content/uploads/2015/01/ReachOut.com-Crossroads-Report-2014.pdf (accessed on 2 July 2017).

16. Paxton, R.; Shrubb, S.; Griffiths, H.; Cameron, L.; Maunder, L. Tiered approach: Matching mental health services to needs. *J. Ment. Health* **2000**, *9*, 137–144.

17. World Health Organization. Comprehensive Mental Health Action Plan 2013–2020. Available online: http://www.who.int/entity/mental_health/action_plan_2013/en/index.html (accessed on 4 July 2017).

18. Simmonds, S.; Coid, J.; Joseph, P.; Marriott, S.; Tyrer, P. Community mental health team management in severe mental illness: A systematic review. *Br. J. Psychiatry* **2001**, *178*, 497–502. [CrossRef] [PubMed]

19. Ng, C.; Herrman, H.; Chiu, E.; Singh, B. Community mental health care in the Asia-Pacific region: Using current best-practice models to inform future policy. *World Psychiatry* **2009**, *8*, 49–55. [CrossRef] [PubMed]

20. Social Welfare Department (The Government of the Hong Kong Special Administrative Region). Integrated Community Center for Mental Wellness (ICCMW). Available online: http://www.swd.gov.hk/en/index/site_pubsvc/page_rehab/sub_listofserv/id_iccmw/ (accessed on 19 June 2017).

21. Hong, S.D. Community mental health system for children and adolescents in Korea. *Psychiatry Investig.* **2006**, *3*, 32–38.

22. SG Enable. Early Intervention Program for Infants & Children (EIPIC). Available online: https://www.sgenable.sg/Pages/content.aspx?path=/for-children/early-intervention-program-for-infants-children-eipic (accessed on 5 July 2017).

23. McGorry, P.; Bates, T.; Birchwood, M. Designing youth mental health services for the 21st century: Examples from Australia, Ireland and the UK. *Br. J. Psychiatry* **2013**, *202*, s30–s35. [CrossRef] [PubMed]

24. Muir, K.; McDermott, S.; Gendera, S.; Flaxman, S.; Patulny, R.; Sitek, T.; Abello, D.; Oprea, I.; Katz, I. *Independent Evaluation of Headspace: The National Youth Mental Health Foundation: Interim Evaluation Report*; Social Policy Research Centre: Sydney, Australia, June 2009.

25. ReachOut. What you Need to Know about Youth Mental Health in Regional Australia. Available online: https://about.au.reachout.com/what-you-need-to-know-about-youth-mental-health-in-regional-australia-2017/ (accessed on 2 July 2017).

26. Chong, S.A.; Abdin, E.; Sherbourne, C.; Vaingankar, J.; Heng, D.; Yap, M.; Subramaniam, M. Treatment gap in common mental disorders: The Singapore perspective. *Epidemiol. Psychiatr. Sci.* **2012**, *21*, 195–202. [CrossRef] [PubMed]

27. Xie, Y.; Boon, J.; Sim, W.H.; Fung, D. A Singapore model-REACH. In *School Mental Health: Global Challenges and Opportunities*; Kutcher, S., Wei, Y., Weist, M.D., Eds.; Cambridge University Press: Cambridge, UK, 2015; pp. 202–217.

28. Ow, R. Mental health care: The Singapore context. *Asia Pac. J. Soc. Work Dev.* **1998**, *8*, 120–130. [CrossRef]

29. Ministry of Health Singapore. Suicide Prevention. Available online: https://www.moh.gov.sg/content/moh_web/home/pressRoom/Parliamentary_QA/2016/suicide-prevention.html (accessed on 26 September 2017).

30. Clinical Global Impression. *ECDEU Assessment Manual for Psychopharmacology (revised)*; Guy, W., Ed.; National Institute of Mental Health: Rockville, MD, USA, 1976; pp. 217–221.

31. Goodman, R. The Strengths and Difficulties Questionnaire: A research note. *J. Child. Psychol. Psychiatry* **1997**, *38*, 581–586. [CrossRef] [PubMed]

32. Cai, S.Y.; Fung, D.S.S. Community mental health as a population-based mental health approach. *Isr. J. Psychiatry Relat. Sci.* **2016**, *53*, 33–39.

33. Fung, D.; Chan, M.C.; Koh, D.; Cai, S.; Wee, H.L. The cost effectiveness of a community mental health service for children and adolescents in Singapore. *J. Ment. Health Policy Econ.* **2014**, *17*, S6.

34. Becker, A.E.; Kleinman, A. Mental health and the global agenda. *N. Engl. J. Med.* **2013**, *369*, 66–73. [CrossRef] [PubMed]

35. Webster-Stratton, C. *The Incredible Years: A Trouble-Shooting Guide for Parents of Children Aged 3–8*. The Umbrella Press: Toronto, ON, Canada, 1997.

36. Sanders, M.R.; Mazzucchelli, T.G.; Studman, L.J. *Facilitator's Manual for Group Stepping Stones Triple P for Families with a Child Who Has a Disability*. Triple P International: Brisbane, Australia, 2009.

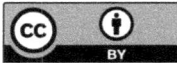

brain
sciences

MDPI

Commentary

A Diagnosis of Denial: How Mental Health Classification Systems Have Struggled to Recognise Family Violence as a Serious Risk Factor in the Development of Mental Health Issues for Infants, Children, Adolescents and Adults

Wendy Bunston [1,2,*], Candice Franich-Ray [3,4,5] and Sara Tatlow [3]

1   Wb Training and Consultancy, P.O. Box 750, Moonee Ponds 3039, Victoria, Australia
2   La Trobe University, Bundoora 3086, Victoria, Australia
3   Mental Health, The Royal Children's Hospital, 50 Flemington Road, Parkville 3052, Victoria, Australia;
     candice.franichray@rch.org.au (C.F.-R.); sara.tatlow@rch.org.au (S.T.)
4   The Murdoch Childrens Research Institute, Flemington Road, Parkville 3052, Victoria, Australia
5   Department of Paediatrics, The University of Melbourne; Level 2 West Building,
     The Royal Children's Hospital, 50 Flemington Street, Parkville 3052, Victoria, Australia
*   Correspondence: wendy.bunston@bigpond.com; Tel.: +61-400-150-090

Received: 31 July 2017; Accepted: 10 October 2017; Published: 17 October 2017

Abstract: Child and adolescent mental health services (CAMHS) routinely overlook assessing for, and providing treatment to, infants and children living with family violence, despite family violence being declared endemic across the globe. As contemporary neuro-developmental research recognises the harm of being exposed to early relational trauma, key international diagnostic texts such as the DSM-5 and ICD-10 struggle to acknowledge or appreciate the relational complexities inherent in addressing family violence and its impacts during childhood. These key texts directly influence thinking, funding and research imperatives in adult services as well as CAMHS, however, they rarely reference family violence. Their emphasis is to pathologise conditions over exploring causality which may be attributable to relational violence. Consequently, CAMHS can miss important indicators of family violence, misdiagnose disorders and unwittingly, not address unacceptable risks in the child's caregiving environment. Notwithstanding urgent safety concerns, ongoing exposure to family violence significantly heightens the development of mental illness amongst children. CAMHS providers cannot and should not rely on current diagnostic manuals alone. They need to act now to see family violence as a significant and important risk factor to mental health and to treat its impacts on children before these develop into enduring neurological difficulties.

Keywords: infants; children; adolescents; family violence; mental health treatment; diagnostic classification of disorders; DSM-5; ICD-10; DC:0-5; CAMHS

1. Introduction

The prevalence of violence within families is considered to be at endemic levels across the world [1–3]. Relational trauma and exposure to toxic stress—in utero and perinatally—has been shown to have enduring and detrimental impacts across development within the early years, childhood, and beyond, significantly increasing the development of mental health disorders [4]. This invited paper provides a commentary on the misalignment between current knowledge regarding early brain development and the application of this knowledge in key mental health diagnostic texts in determining, or failing to determine, responses to children impacted by familial violence. It is standard practice across western child and adolescent mental health services to use the criterion of two significant classification and diagnostic manuals in their assessment and treatment plans for children and young people. These two texts are the DSM-5 (Diagnostic and Statistical Manual of Mental Disorders) produced by the American Psychiatric Association [5], and the ICD-10 (International Statistical Classification of Diseases and Related Health Problems) produced by the World Health Organisation [6].

A review was undertaken systematically to ascertain how family violence is referred to within the DSM-5 and the ICD-10. The outcome of these reviews is provided. An additional review was also undertaken of a third important classification manual used when working within infant mental health, the DC:0-5 (Diagnostic Classification of Mental Health and Developmental Disorders of Infancy and Early Childhood) [7]. This small, lesser known, but significant classification manual was developed by workers in the field of infant mental health to help Child and Adolescent Mental Health Services (CAMHS) think about the early experience of infants and young children. The focus of this third text is on classifying behaviours consistent with diagnoses in the DSM-5 and ICD-10 but where early onset is indicated [7]. The results of the review of these three diagnostic classification manuals are provided and the omission of any clear references to family violence within the reviews discussed. The paper concludes that CAMHS, adult mental health services and indeed the infants, children and families impacted by family violence, cannot afford to wait for traditional mental health classification manuals to adequately capture and report on the complexities and risk factors associated with family violence. CAMHS needs to recognise and respond to the scientific research and prevalence evidence now to offer appropriate and timely treatment responses for children. Furthermore, adult mental health services need to name and assess for family violence, remaining cognisant of the fact that the children of their patients who experience family violence are likely to also be victims of that violence.

1.1. Prevalence, Causes and Impacts of Family Violence

Whilst debate exists around defining family violence, the distinction is that "in contrast to other forms of violence ... relationships usually exist between family violence victims and perpetrators prior to, during, and after violent incidents" [8] (p. 599). Despite differences in terminology including "domestic violence", "intimate partner violence" (IPV), "wife battering", "violence against women and children" [8–13] there is consensus across the globe that violence within intimate relationships has reached endemic proportions [2,3,10,14–19]. The research to date overwhelmingly identifies violence, and/or homicide, which occurs within intimate partner relationships as gendered, with women most at risk of harm by their male partners [3,20]. According to the UN Women's Council, "One in three women will experience some form of physical and/or sexual violence in her lifetime" [20] (p. 16). This does not mean that men themselves do not experience violence within heterosexual interpersonal relationships [15,21–23], nor that violence is not experienced within same sex relationships [24–26].

Explanations for what causes violence within families remains complex, with societal attitudes, gender and cultural inequalities, economic pressures and intergenerational transmission of interpersonal violence often cited as significant contributors [10,13,27,28]. Homelessness, alcohol and substance abuse issues, as well as mental health difficulties are also identified as serious risk factors associated with the prevalence of family violence [10,27,29–34]. The costs of family violence to society is monumental. Notwithstanding the social and health implications for the individual, the family and the community, the economic costs to societies across the globe are almost incalculable. Various countries across the world have estimated that economic costs of violence against women and their children to be in the billions [11,35–39]. The use of violence within any intimate relationships is increasingly condemned in most societies today [3]. The impact of family violence on infants, children and adolescents is receiving increasing attention and the inherent detrimental implications for their health and wellbeing over time is becoming better understood [40–46]. Whether infants, children and adolescents reside in a family where their parent is heterosexual, or same-sex, or caregivers are extended family members or otherwise, living with family violence exposes them to an unacceptable risk of harm [3,29,35,47,48].

1.2. Infants, Children's and Adolescent's Exposure to Violence

Measuring the number of infants, children and adolescent's present and/or as the direct victim of family violence has been difficult to ascertain. This is often due to a failure to collect reliable data specific to children [44]. Nevertheless, Lieberman, Chu, Van Horn and Harris [43] contend that empirical evidence demonstrates that children under five are more likely than older children to be exposed to trauma, including that which is caused by domestic violence. This is because younger children, and infants in particular, are more likely to be in the immediate care of, or in close proximity to their mothers during violent episodes perpetrated by partners [49]. The younger the child the less capacity they have to protect themselves, flee the violence or be in other environments when violence occurs, such as school, after school care etc. Research has indicated that some women become the victims of violence once they fall pregnant, with the father of the baby more commonly, though not exclusively, identified as the perpetrator [50,51]. Violence during pregnancy increases the risk of infant mortality, premature births and low birth weights [52–56]. In teenage pregnancy, the prevalence of partner violence and increased risks to mother and infant are particularly high [53,57–59]. It is estimated that 1 in 4 children will be exposed to family violence in their lifetime [29,47,60]. Australian women reported children being present up to 31% of the time during episodes of violence by their partners [61]. A survey conducted across the European Union reported that 73% of women who had experienced partner violence believed their children were aware of the violence [10].

The World Health Organisation (WHO) states that violence is preventable and has identified six clear strategies to effect this. The first two of these imperatives directly concern the early years and involve "developing safe, stable and nurturing relationships between children and their parents and caregivers" and "developing life skills in children and adolescents" [3] (p.viii). The United States National Intimate Partner and Sexual Violence Survey agrees. They state that the key to prevention may be through developing "Strategies that support the development of safe, stable, nurturing relationships and environments for parents or caregivers and their children" [15] (p.5). The sheer volume of infants, children and adolescents, who with their mothers and primary caregivers are exposed to family violence, warrants a comprehensive treatment response by CAMHS.

1.3. Research on How Family Violence and Relational Trauma Impacts Infant and Child Development

Family violence creates relational trauma for all family members, as it disrupts and disturbs all relationships within the family, not just the relationship between warring parents/adults. The quality and continuity of early caregiving experiences has been proven to be crucial to the development of social, emotional, physical and mental health in children [62–69]. Early infant/parent relationship research is often commonly understood in terms of the attachment the infant develops with their primary caregiver, and how this then directly impacts the infant's neurological, physiological, psychological and emotional development [70–75]. Schwerdtfeger and Goff [76] found that where expectant mothers had a history of interpersonal trauma they "reported significantly higher trauma symptoms and lower prenatal attachment than those who reported no history of interpersonal trauma" (p. 46). Research into exposure to domestic violence during pregnancy was also found to negatively impact the way mothers' see their infant [77,78]. Furthermore, ongoing exposure to family violence was associated with the child developing an insecure attachment with their mother by the age of four [79–81]. Exposure to family violence creates relational ruptures which can interrupt the healthy formation of safe and reliable bonds between children and their parent/s [78,79]. This impacts subsequent social relationships, and produces adult attachment behaviours including an oversensitivity to rejection, avoidant and ambivalent patterns of relating and increased risk of replicating violence in intimate relationships [82–84]. Attachment theory pioneer John Bowlby considered family violence a "disorder of attachment" [85]. He believed enormous psychological damage was done to the child and the family system, and was puzzled as to why "family violence as a causal factor in psychiatry should have been so neglected" (p. 9).

Where the infant or very young child is traumatised by the violence of one or both parents and/or caregivers there is little to nowhere for the infant or young child to seek safety and protection; as they are dependent on the very caregiving system which is generating the trauma [82,86–89]. Early exposure to interpersonal trauma such as family violence impacts the emerging subjectivity of the infant and impinges negatively on their developing mental states, capacity for affect regulation and has implications for their later forming executive functioning [40,90–95]. Levendosky, Bogat and Martinez-Torteya [42] found that "children are affected by the IPV they witness and often show a traumatic response. The expression of traumatic symptoms is likely to increases as children age; this is consistent with the trajectory of other anxiety disorders and internalising disorders generally" (p. 195). Thus, exposure to violence from birth impacts the developing regulatory capacities of the infant, with increasing socioemotional difficulties being displayed by 12 months [91]. Children up to the age of 8 years have been found to have lower cognitive scores than their peers who were not exposed to family violence [40]. In particular, internalising and externalising difficulties become more apparent for children as they approach school age and beyond, evidenced through anxious, avoidant and/or disruptive behaviours [42,92]. Children and adolescents exposed to ongoing family violence are increasingly recognised within the literature as manifesting symptoms consistent with Post Traumatic Stress Disorder (PTSD) and other psychiatric disorders [46,96–100].

1.4. The Science of Brain Development

Research into the impacts of trauma on the developing brain has been significant [4,63,64,74,86,101–103]. The developing infant brain is decidedly 'experience dependent' and shaped by the caregiving environment [4,62,104]. "Infants and young children exposed to chronic stress or traumas may have increased levels of the stress hormones cortisol, epinephrine and norepinephrine; chronic high levels of these hormones can have negative effects on emotional regulation, cognitive development, and brain development" [4] (p. 386). Further, crucial to healthy infant development is the regulatory role played by the hypothalamic-pituitary-adrenal (HPA) axis and the associated neuroendocrine responses to stress [105]. Disturbances in the functioning of the HPA axis have been found to have particular implications for the development of neuropsychiatric conditions [106]. In addition, ongoing and significant early relational trauma can impact synaptic growth, reduce hippocampal, cerebellar, and corpus callosum volume, as well as risk damaging limbic regions and the prefrontal cortex; deficits consistent with paediatric posttraumatic stress disorder [107].

Direct research on how family violence impacts the infant brain has been inferred from research into the impact of trauma and stress on the developing brain generally [4,95,103]. However, research using neuroimaging with mothers who have been diagnosed with interpersonal violence related PTSD has found their capacity to read their infants social cues is limited [108]. It is the caregiving relationship that operates as the primary organiser in how the infant brain develops. Where this is impacted by the mother's own trauma [73,86,109] and further where the infant is a witness "it is likely that exposure to IPV can impact a very young child's neurological development in detrimental ways that in turn can impact other domains of development" [4] (p. 834). Neuroimaging of infants during ordinary sleep found that even exposure to angry verbal conflict alone elicited heightened responses in the brain regions concerned with emotional regulation and processing, implying that even moderate stress can impact infant brain functioning [110]. There is little doubt that acute, ongoing stress affects neural circuity, and no more so than during the early years [74,95,101,111–113]. In light of the mounting evidence regarding the impacts of family violence on infants, children and adolescents, how mental health services assess and treat these impacts is a key concern.

2. Combined Methods and Results

2.1. Referencing Violence within DSM-5

The DSM-5 is nearly 1000 pages long and is separated into three different sections and an appendix. The principal section is Section II, which is 696 pages and lists all mental disorder classifications. This section includes 21 overarching 'diagnostic categories' and an additional section of conditions that may be clinically relevant but are not mental disorders. It explains the criteria for these categories and supplies their corresponding ICD-9 and ICD-10 codes.

Section II: Diagnostic Criteria and Codes was reviewed systematically for any mention of the terms "family violence", "domestic violence", "interpersonal violence" and "partner violence". Further, any specific reference of the word "violence" was examined and if there was any indication that this could refer to being a victim or perpetrator of family violence this was included (note, however, that terms such as "sexual violence" and "physical violence" in the context of child abuse were excluded unless it was specific to a family violence context). "Community violence" also emerged, however, this term was excluded from the review as it was felt to reflect violence in the wider community rather than within the family. Additional, potentially related terms such as "adverse events" and "trauma" were also reviewed to establish any association with family violence. During the initial review process, mention of "spouse/spousal beating" also emerged as a descriptor which could be appropriately defined as linking with the term "family violence". This term was then added to the search. The results can be found in Table 1 below. Terms relating to "Abuse" (including "childhood abuse", "physical abuse", "sexual abuse", "neglect" and "maltreatment") were also systematically reviewed. Although they are also significant stressors impacting mental health they were not included in the final table of findings or the discussion presented below as a connection to family violence was not specified.

Section II concludes with a final 'catch-all' category titled "Other Conditions That May Be a Focus of Clinical Attention" [5] and it is noted in the text that these conditions are not mental disorders but "may affect the patient's care" (For the sake of continuity, the word "patient" will be used forthwith over other possible descriptors such as "consumer" or "client".) (p. 715) and can be coded "if it is a reason for the current visit or helps to explain the need for a test, procedure, or treatment" (p. 715). It is here that there is more attention to family violence related issues, specifically with regards to violence occurring within intimate (adult) relationships. Spouse or Partner Violence either Physical or Sexual as well as Spouse or Partner Neglect and Spouse or Partner Abuse Psychological are included in this section and signify whether the patient is or has been a victim of intimate partner violence, or, has been a perpetrator and whether it is either confirmed or suspected. In Spouse or Partner Violence, a description is given which specifies events that have occurred over the past year [5], however, the codes attached to this description simply states "personal history (past history) of spouse or partner violence..." (p. 720) making it unclear to the reader if this acknowledges any possible long term impacts on the individual. There is also no mention, where violence has occurred over the past year, of any children of the patient being potentially impacted by this very same violence.

The term "family violence" was not mentioned at all in the mental disorders categories in Section II of the DMS-5. The term "partner violence" was, however, included in the diagnostic criteria for three disorders in the Sexual Dysfunction category and in the Other Conditions That May Be a Focus of Clinical Attention category. "Domestic violence", "interpersonal violence", "violence" and "spouse/spousal beating" were mentioned an additional eleven times with two being that of a possible perpetrator. These were in the following disorders: PTSD; Acute Stress Disorder; Depersonalization/Derealisation Disorder; Somatic Symptoms and Related Disorders; Conduct Disorder; and Antisocial Personality Disorder.

Table 1. Frequency of the terms "family violence", "domestic violence", "interpersonal violence", "partner violence", "violence", "spouse/spousal beating", "adverse" and "trauma/tic" in the context of family violence and events experienced or perpetrated in the DSM 5 Section II.

Diagnostic Category DSM-5	Number of Times the Following Terms Are Referred to in Text				Direct Quote of the Term from the Text
	"Violence" Experienced[1]	"Spouse/Spousal Beating"	"Adverse" Events Experienced	"Trauma/Tic" Events Experienced	
Neurodevelopmental Disorders	0	0	0	0	
Schizophrenia Spectrum and Other Psychotic Disorders	0	0	0	0	
Bipolar and Related Disorders	0	0	0	0	
Depressive Disorders	0	0	1	1	Major Depressive Disorder: "Adverse childhood experiences, particularly when there are multiple experiences of diverse types, constitute a set of potent risk factors for major depressive disorder. . . " p. 166 Premenstrual Dysphoric Disorder: "Environmental factors associated with the expression of premenstrual dysphoric disorder include . . . history of interpersonal trauma..." p. 173
Anxiety Disorders	0	0	0	0	
Obsessive-Compulsive and Related Disorders	0	0	0	2	Obsessive Compulsive Disorder: "Physical and sexual abuse in childhood and other stressful or traumatic events have been associated with an increased risk for developing OCD" p. 239 Hoarding Disorder: "Individuals with hoarding disorder often retrospectively report stressful and traumatic life events preceding the onset of the disorder or causing an exacerbation" p. 249
Trauma- and Stressor-Related Disorders	6	0	0	DC[2]	'Traumatic' was included repetitively in the diagnostic criteria for Posttraumatic Stress Disorder and Acute Stress Disorder[3] Posttraumatic Stress Disorder: (i) "Witnessed events include . . . domestic violence . . . " p. 274 (ii) "Children may experience co-occurring traumas (e.g., physical abuse, witnessing domestic violence) and in chronic circumstances may not be able to identify onset of symptomatology" p. 277 (iii) "Peritraumatic Factors . . . These include . . . interpersonal violence (particularly trauma perpetrated by a caregiver or involving a witnessed threat to a caregiver in children)" p. 278 (iv) "At least some of the increased risk for PTSD in females appears to be attributable to a greater likelihood of exposure to traumatic events, such as rape, and other forms of interpersonal violence . . . " p. 278 Acute Stress Disorder: (i) "Witnessed events include . . . severe domestic violence..." p. 282 (ii) "The increased risk for the disorder in females may be attributable in part to a greater likelihood of exposure to the types of traumatic events with a high conditional risk for acute stress disorder, such as rape and other interpersonal violence" p. 285

Table 1. *Cont.*

Diagnostic Category DSM-5	Number of Times the Following Terms Are Referred to in Text				Direct Quote of the Term from the Text
	"Violence" Experienced [1]	"Spouse/Spousal Beating"	"Adverse" Events Experienced	"Trauma/Tic" Events Experienced	
Dissociative Disorders	2	0	1	DC	Dissociative Amnesia [3]: "Dissociative amnesia is more likely to occur with (1) a greater number of adverse childhood experiences, particularly physical and/or sexual abuse; (2) interpersonal violence; (3) increased severity, frequency, and violence of the trauma" p. 300 Depersonalization/Derealisation Disorder: "Other stressors can include … witnessing domestic violence … " p. 304
Somatic Symptom and Related Disorders	1	0	0	2	Introduction to Somatic Symptom and Related Disorders: "A number of factors may contribute to somatic symptom and related disorders. These include … early traumatic experiences (e.g., violence, abuse, deprivation) … " p. 310 Conversion Disorder: "Onset may be associated with stress or trauma, either psychological or physical in nature." pp. 319
Feeding and Eating Disorders	0	0	0	0	
Elimination Disorders	0	0	0	0	
Sleep Wake Disorders	0	0	1	2	Nightmare Disorder: (i) "Nightmares occurring after traumatic experiences may replicate the threatening situation ("replicative nightmares"), but most do not" p. 404 (ii) "Individuals who experience nightmares report more frequent past adverse events … but not necessarily trauma" p. 405
Sexual Dysfunctions	DC	0	0	1	Diagnostic Criteria for Female Orgasmic Disorder, Female Sexual Interest/Arousal Disorder and Genito-Pelvic Pain/Penetration Disorder [3] "The sexual dysfunction is not better explained by a nonsexual mental disorder or as a consequence of severe relationship distress (e.g., partner violence) … " pp. 429–440 Male Hypoactive Sexual Desire Disorder: " … trauma resulting from early life experiences must be taken into account in explaining the low desire … " p. 442
Gender Dysphoria	0	0	0	0	
Disruptive, Impulse-Control, and Conduct Disorders	1	0	0	1	Intermittent Explosive Disorder: "Individuals with a history of physical and emotional trauma during the first two decades of life are at increased risk … " p. 467 Conduct Disorder: "When individuals with conduct disorder reach adulthood, symptoms of aggression, property destruction, deceitfulness, and rule violation, including violence against co-workers, partners, and children, may be exhibited in the workplace and the home … " p. 473
Substance-Related and Addictive Disorders	0	0	0	2	Inhalant Use Disorder: "Childhood maltreatment or trauma also is associated with youthful progression from inhalant non-use to inhalant use disorder" p. 536 Other (or unknown) Substance Use Disorder: "Risk and prognostic factors for other (or unknown) substance use disorders are thought to be similar to those for most substance use disorders and include … childhood maltreatment or trauma…" p. 580

Table 1. *Cont.*

Diagnostic Category DSM-5	Number of Times the Following Terms Are Referred to in Text				Direct Quote of the Term from the Text
	"Violence" Experienced [1]	"Spouse/Spousal Beating"	"Adverse" Events Experienced	"Trauma/Tic" Events Experienced	
Neurocognitive Disorders	0	0	0	0	
Personality Disorders	0	1	0	0	Antisocial personality disorder "Individuals with antisocial personality disorder tend to be irritable and aggressive and may repeatedly get into physical fights or commit acts of physical assault (including spouse beating or child beating)" p. 660
Paraphilic Disorders	0	0	0	0	
Other Mental Disorders	0	0	0	0	
Medication-Induced Movement Disorders and Other Adverse Effects of Medication	0	0	0	0	
Other Conditions That May Be a Focus of Clinical Attention [4]	DC	0	0	1	Adult Maltreatment and Neglect Problems (1) Spouse or Partner Violence, Physical: "This category should be used when non-accidental acts of physical force that result, or have reasonable potential to result, in physical harm to an intimate partner or that evoke significant fear in the partner that have occurred during the past year..." p. 720 (2) Spouse of Partner Violence, Sexual: "This category should be used when forced or coerced sexual acts with an intimate partner have occurred during the past year..." p. 720 Housing Problems, Homelessness: "An individual is considered to be homeless if his or her primary night-time residence is a homeless shelter, a warming shelter, a domestic violence shelter..." p. 723 Other Personal History of Psychological Trauma p. 726
Total [5]	10	1	3	12	
Total DC	2	0	0	2	

[1] The following terms were included: "family violence", "domestic violence", "interpersonal violence", "partner violence", "violence" (when in context of family violence); [2] DC: Term included in the Diagnostic Criteria; [3] No quote or reduced quotes have been included as there are multiple instances of the term as it is part of the diagnostic criteria; [4] Note these are not mental disorders but were included in Section II of the DSM-5; [5] DC are not included in the overall frequency total but a frequency of DC is reported in "Total DC".

As there are 152 mental disorders listed in the DSM-5 (excluding disorders that are 'Not Otherwise specified' or 'Other specified/unspecified'), [5,114] there are many disorders where family violence could readily have been included yet was not. In particular, it was surprising that there were no links made to interpersonal or family violence as a risk factor in the following disorders given that the research suggests otherwise: Schizophrenia Spectrum and Other Psychotic Disorders [115–117], Depressive Disorders [118–121], Anxiety Disorders [118,121], Substance-Related and Addictive Disorders [34,122–125], Personality Disorders [126,127]. However, this absence of referring to family or interpersonal violence may also be attributable to the use of terminology within the DSM-5 itself. For example, within Anxiety Disorders imprecise and broad terms were used. The term "life stress" was referred to in Separation Anxiety Disorder; "interpersonal stressors" were referred to in Panic Disorder; the term "negative events in childhood" for Agoraphobia and "stressful life situations" was mentioned in Rumination Disorder. That there is no specific mention of family, domestic or interpersonal violence in childhood within Anxiety Disorders, however, is perplexing given the avalanche of research identifying anxiety in children exposed to family violence [4,42,43,45,46,94–96,99,128].

When the terms "domestic violence", "interpersonal violence", "partner violence", "violence", "adverse" and "trauma" were mentioned they were usually referred to in the Risk and Prognostic Factors Section of each disorder. This section is well suited to including family violence. When completing the review of the text it was noted that the Risk and Prognostic Factors Section was not the same for different diagnostic categories with assorted terminology used, distinct focuses and varying depth of description. It is possible that this reflects the different working groups that developed the current DSM-5 [5]. Where "partner violence" was mentioned in three disorders of Sexual Dysfunction these were related to female specific disorders only, with no references made to partner violence within the male specific sexual disorders. Conduct Disorder and Antisocial Personality Disorders were the only disorders where there was a reference to perpetrating family violence. These were the only times children and spouses were explicitly written about as being relationally impacted by the violent actions of the patient. This is surprising given current good practice requires that all family members, whether victims or perpetrators, and their children, receive timely and appropriate support and treatment to address family violence and its impacts [129].

It needs to be acknowledged that there may be other possible ways of describing family violence which were not elicited by this review. The term "spouse beating", as already mentioned, emerged only whilst searching for other possible ways of describing family violence. Terms which may be referred to as perpetrating an "assault" or "violent acts/behaviour" towards others were not included in this review. Poor terminology and a lack of referring to family members impacted by an "assault" or "violent acts/behaviour" suggests that this is an area needing urgent attention in future revisions. Similarly, not included enough was the "potential" for perpetrating violence against a family member. This was implied in Alcohol Use Disorder [5] and is interesting to note: "individuals with an alcohol use disorder may continue to consume alcohol despite the knowledge that continued consumption poses significant physical (e.g., blackouts, liver disease), psychological (e.g., depression), social, or interpersonal problems (e.g., violent arguments with spouse while intoxicated, child abuse)" (p. 492).

2.2. Referencing Violence within ICD-10

ICD-10 [6] is a manual used worldwide to classify physical and mental diagnoses and to identify factors, such as social circumstances, which may impact them. The World Health Organization states the ICD-10 (in the Purpose and Uses section online) "is the foundation for the identification of health trends and statistics globally, and the international standard for reporting diseases and health conditions. It is the diagnostic classification standard for all clinical and research purposes" [6]. The ICD has been revised several times, with the most recent being the ICD-10 Version: 2016. Used for recording, analysing, interpreting and comparing mortality and morbidity data worldwide, the ICD-10 provides alphanumeric code for disease and other health problems. This system allows for easy storage and retrieval of this data for research purposes [130].

The ICD-10 2016 online edition Section V Mental and behavioural disorders and Section XXI Factors influencing health status and contact with health services was systematically reviewed for any mention of the terms "family violence", "domestic violence", "interpersonal violence", "partner violence", "violence", "spouse/spousal beating", "adverse" and "trauma/tic". The same method of searching as for the DSM-5 was used for the ICD-10. See DSM-5 section for details. The results can be found in Table 2 below.

The term "family violence" does not appear anywhere in the ICD-10. The term "severe interpersonal violence" is mentioned under Problems in Relationship with Spouse or Partner suggesting that only "severe" interpersonal violence is considered important. This reference to interpersonal violence does not include any mention of infants, children and adolescents who may witness or be impacted by this discord. The term "violence" is mentioned under Problems related to alleged Physical Abuse of Child, however these references are relegated to a section of the ICD-10 which is concerned not with the coding of mental disorder specific criterion, but the description of additional factors which might impact the key mental disorder coding criteria. The term "assault" is used in Section XX—External Causes of Morbidity and Mortality to provide specific examples of injury to another person made and the term "abuse" is mentioned under Maltreatment Syndromes in Section XIX—Injury, Poisoning and Certain Other Consequences of External Causes, in reference to physical, sexual and childhood abuse. Surprisingly, these also do not mention family violence and its role in both abuse and assault. The term "serious mishandling" is mentioned in the criteria for Reactive Attachment Disorder of Childhood, however, this term is not fully explained and no link to family violence is made. When the additional terms of "adverse" and "trauma" were searched, two additional mentions were found. "Adverse experiences" are mentioned in Dissocial Personality Disorder whilst "trauma" is mentioned in the criteria for Post-Traumatic Stress Disorder. However, neither mention "family nor interpersonal violence" as a source of the trauma or adversity experienced.

As with the DSM-5, there are many other diagnostic categories in which family violence could realistically and appropriately have been mentioned, but was excluded from the ICD-10. Within the chapter relating specifically to mental health, Chapter V Mental and Behavioural Disorders, domestic violence was omitted from every diagnosis. This is surprising given the plethora of research suggesting more than a strong correlation between domestic violence and the development of mental health disorders [129,131–137]. Although not mental health specific, it was also noted that domestic violence could have also been mentioned as a risk factor for complications under Chapter XV Pregnancy, Childbirth and the Puerperium; throughout Chapter XVI—Certain Conditions Originating in the Perinatal Period; Chapter XIX Injury, Poisoning and Certain Other Consequences of External Causes; and Chapter XX External Causes of Morbidity and Mortality. Furthermore, although mentioned twice (see Table 2 for details), domestic violence could have reasonably been mentioned throughout Chapter XXI Factors Influencing Health Status and Contact with Health Services.

Table 2. Frequency of the terms "family violence", "domestic violence", "interpersonal violence", "partner violence", "violence", "spouse/spousal beating", "adverse" and "trauma/tic" in the context of family violence and events experienced or perpetrated in the ICD-10 2016 (online) Edition [6].

Section	Diagnostic Categories	Number of Times the Following Terms Are Referred to in Text				Direct Quote of the Term from the Text
		"Violence" Experienced [1]	"Spouse/Spousal Beating"	"Adverse" Events Experienced	"Trauma/Tic" Events Experienced	
Section V—Mental and Behavioural disorders						
	Organic, including symptomatic, mental disorders	0	0	0	0	
	Mental and behavioural disorders due to psychoactive substance use	0	0	0	0	
	Schizophrenia	0	0	0	0	
	Schizotypal disorder	0	0	0	0	
	Persistent delusional disorder	0	0	0	0	
	Acute and transient psychotic disorders	0	0	0	0	
	Induced delusional disorder	0	0	0	0	
	Schizoaffective disorders	0	0	0	0	
	other nonorganic psychotic disorders	0	0	0	0	
	Unspecified nonorganic disorders	0	0	0	0	
	Mood (affective) disorders	0	0	0	0	
	Neurotic, stress-related and somatoform disorders	0	0	0	DC [2]	F43.1 PTSD " ... Typical features include episodes of repeated reliving of the trauma in intrusive memories ("flashbacks"), dreams or nightmares, occurring against the persisting background of a sense of "numbness" and emotional blunting, detachment from other people, unresponsiveness to surroundings, anhedonia, and avoidance of activities and situations reminiscent of the trauma ... The onset follows the trauma with a latency period that may range from a few weeks to months ... "
	Behavioural syndromes associated with physiological disturbances and physical factors	0	0	0	0	
	Disorders of adult personality and behaviour	0	0	0	0	
	Mental retardation	0	0	0	0	
	Disorders of psychological development	0	0	0	0	
	Behavioural and emotional disorders with onset usually occurring in childhood and adolescence	0	0	0	0	
	Unspecified mental disorder	0	0	0	0	

Table 2. *Cont.*

Section	Diagnostic Categories	Number of Times the Following Terms Are Referred to in Text				Direct Quote of the Term from the Text
		"Violence" Experienced [1]	"Spouse/Spousal Beating"	"Adverse" Events Experienced	"Trauma/Tic" Events Experienced	
Section XXI actors influencing health status and contact with health services						
	Persons encountering health services for examination and investigation	0	0	0	0	
	Persons with potential health hazards related to communicable diseases	0	0	0	0	
	Persons encountering health services in circumstances related to reproduction	0	0	0	0	
	Persons encountering health services for specific procedures and health care	0	0	0	0	
	Persons with potential health hazards related to socioeconomic and psychosocial circumstances	0	0	0	0	
	Persons encountering health services in other circumstances	0	0	0	0	
	Persons with potential health hazards related to family and personal history and certain conditions influencing health status	DC	0	0	0	Z63.0 Problems in relationship with spouse or partner: "Discord between partners resulting in severe or prolonged loss of control, in generalization of hostile or critical feelings or in a persisting atmosphere of severe interpersonal violence (hitting or striking)"
Total [3]		0	0	1	0	
Total DC		1	0	0	1	

[1] The following terms were included: "family violence", "domestic violence", "interpersonal violence", "partner violence", "violence" (when in context of family violence); [2] DC: Term included in the Diagnostic Criteria; [3] DC are not included in the overall frequency total but a frequency of DC is reported in "Total DC".

2.3. Mental Illness in Children and the DC:0-5

Previously known as the DC:0-3 [138], the expanded DC:0-5 was released in 2016 and included a new classification of specific Relationship Disorders in Axis I [7]. This encourages the recognition that difficulties can lay outside of the child, and that relational complexities can occur between one caregiver and the infant/child rather than as a feature of the infant or child's relationships across all their significant relationships. The DC:0-5 is a 212 page diagnostic classification manual for infants and young children produced by Zero To Three in Washington [7]. The DC:0-5 is a multi-axial system with; Axis I providing clinical diagnoses (grouped into eight categories), Axis II providing the relational context, Axis III providing physical health conditions and considerations, Axis IV psychosocial stressors and Axis V developmental competence. The use of a multi-axial diagnostic system can assist the reader in considering the context around the individual rather than just focusing on the pathology. The DC:0-5 is developmentally sensitive and incorporates the need to assess for risk, as well as protective factors. It is cognisant of the importance of considering the growing infant and young child's context, culture and relationships in impacting on emerging mental health disorders. Furthermore, as a mental health and developmental disorders manual for early childhood [7], it also readily acknowledges that "behaviours of infants/young children may differ systematically with different caregivers . . . There are also numerous case reports of symptomatic behaviour in one caregiving relationship that does not generalise to other relationships" (p. 134).

Review of Axis I was conducted using the same systematic method as the DSM-5 and ICD-10. See Table 3 for results.

The inclusion of Relationship Disorders [7] in Axis I and Axis II Relational Context, is intended to encourage practitioners to assess for "cumulative severity of stresses" including "noting their duration and severity" (p. 154). Axis IV Psychosocial Stressors includes the Psychosocial and Environmental Stressor Checklist with 77 different possible stressors listed for clinicians to be aware of when diagnosing mental health disorders. In the introduction section of this Axis domestic violence has been mentioned: "Psychosocial stressors for an infant/young child include acute events and enduring circumstances. Examples of the latter include poverty and domestic violence" [7] (p. 153). In the list "domestic violence" features as one of multiple possible stressors that need to be assessed. Unfortunately, the checklist is designed to measure the number of co-occurring stresses as more "predictive of subsequent maladaptation than any specific stressors" [7] (p. 153). While domestic violence is cited as an example of an enduring psychosocial stressor, its impacts can be understood to be heightened or mitigated by the developmental level of the infant or child, the severity of the violence and the protective buffers offered by the caregivers within that environment "to help the infant/young child understand and cope with the stressor" [7] (p. 153).

As was found with the review of DSM-5 and ICD-10, the DC:0-5 had limited mention of family violence as a risk factor for particular mental disorders. For example, Sensory Over Responsivity Disorder, included "environmental conditions—including lack of movement/tactile stimulation in the early years (e.g., due to being raised in an orphanage, exposure to drugs or prenatal stress, cumulative risk, or community violence—appear to increase risk for Sensory Over-Responsivity Disorder" [7] (p. 441) but made no mention of domestic violence [45,95,110,139]. However, it was specifically mentioned in Anxiety Disorders and Trauma, Stress, and Deprivation Disorders.

Table 3. Frequency of the terms "family violence", "domestic violence", "interpersonal violence", "partner violence", "violence", "spouse/spousal beating", "adverse" and "trauma/tic" in the context of family violence and events experienced or perpetrated in the DC:0-5 Axis I.

Diagnostic Category DC:0-5	Number of Times the Following Terms Are Referred to in Text				Direct Quote of the Term from the Text
	"Violence" Experienced [1]	"Spouse/Spousal Beating"	"Adverse" Events Experienced	"Trauma/Tic" Events Experienced	
Neurodevelopmental Disorders	0	0	1	0	"For example, young children raised in adverse caregiving environments, such as institutions or orphanages, have approximately a fourfold risk of ADHD in early childhood compared with non-maltreated pre-schoolers living in families" p. 28
Sensory Processing Disorders	0	0	0	0	
Anxiety Disorders	1	0	0	1	"Risk factors associated with impairing anxiety in early childhood include … environmental factors (e.g., exposure to violence[2], particularly domestic violence), adverse[2] life experiences (e.g., medical illnesses requiring hospitalizations and procedures) …" p. 56–57 "mutism that presents suddenly after a major traumatic event should be identified as traumatic mutism, not Selective Mutism" p. 60
Mood Disorders	0	0	0	0	
Obsessive Compulsive and Related Disorders	0	0	0	0	
Sleep, Eating, and Crying Disorders	0	0	0	1	"Compared with adults, nightmares in young children can happen more commonly without an identified traumatic exposure, although the social context is important to consider clinically" p. 96
Trauma, Stress, and Deprivation Disorders	DC [3,4]	0	0	DC [4]	"The infant/young child was exposed to significant threat of or actual serious injury, accident, illness, medical trauma, significant loss, disaster, violence (e.g., partner violence, community violence, war or terrorism), or physical/sexual abuse in one or more of the following ways …" p. 115
Relationship Disorders	0	0	0	0	
Total [5]	2	0	1	2	
Total DC	1	0	0	1	

[1] The following terms were included: "family violence", "domestic violence", "interpersonal violence", "partner violence", "violence" (when in context of family violence); [2] "violence" and "adverse" were not counted in these instances as "domestic violence" was mentioned separately so these incidences of "exposure to violence" and "adverse life experiences" were not referring to family violence; [3] DC: Term included in the Diagnostic Criteria; [4] No quote or reduced quotes have been included as there are multiple instances of the term as it is part of the diagnostic criteria; [5] DC are not included in the overall frequency total but a frequency of DC is reported in "Total DC".

3. Discussion

This review found that there was a dearth of references to violence occurring within familial relationships across the DSM-5, the ICD-10 and the DC:0-5. By largely omitting an acknowledgement of family violence as a significant risk factor in the development of multiple mental health disorders the enormity of the problem is effectively denied and the opportunity to offer interventions to address the fallout from family violence is missed. Specifically, this ignores the reality that large numbers of adult patients with mental health problems have previously and may also currently be experiencing family violence. Additionally, these same patients may be parents of children who are also exposed to current violence. In particular, the DSM-5 and ICD-10's failure to recognise the links between early childhood exposure to family violence and mental health disorders, and assessing for current exposure to family violence essentially disappears and therefore disavows the experience of infants, children, adolescents and adults impacted by that violence. By not naming, not seeing and not assessing for family violence, historically or currently, there is no recognition that violence within families impacts all members of that family, no matter their age [140,141]. This averts any need to think about, or take action to intervene now and address the safety needs of the children of the considerable number of adults with mental health disorders who are victims and/or perpetrators of family violence [98,131]. Not considering the children of adult mental health clients who use violence avoids the need to take any action to ensure that those children are safe or to assess their potential need for treatment. Furthermore, the trickledown effect of omitting any significant reference to family violence in adult classification manuals is that within CAMHS, family violence is similarly, often not identified as a serious risk for emerging "mental health problems".

Terminology within both DSM-5 and the ICD-10 was highly problematic. For example, in searching for terms that may point to the incidence of family violence, words such as "assault", "serious mishandling", "adverse events" and "discord" were evident. Their meanings, however, appeared nebulous. The terms were neither fully explained nor the context within which they occurred clearly spelt out. There was also no mention of domestic violence in Section XIX of the ICD-10 which refers to assault as a result of external sources (e.g., drowning, strangulation etc.). Given the reluctance domestic violence victims often have in engaging with services and help seeking and the impacts on physical and mental health [17,118,122,129,142–145], domestic violence, in its various forms (e.g., intergenerational, spousal, family) should all have separate codes in all three manuals with specific examples of what each form of domestic violence means and be mentioned or referred to in the diagnostic criteria for mental health disorders. Additionally, it would be helpful to have specifier codes which allow clinicians to identify/record if the violence is chronic, acute or improving. Doing so would draw attention to the importance of family and domestic violence in assessing and treating patients and acknowledge the impact on the functioning and engagement of the patient. The World Health Organisation (WHO), which produces the ICD-10 [6], is also the very organisation which has produced repeated reports on the endemic of interpersonal violence across the globe [1–3,17]. It would appear judicious for the findings of these WHO produced global reports on interpersonal violence to be meaningfully and responsibly incorporated into the ICD-10, the WHO's international classification manual "for monitoring of the incidence and prevalence of diseases and other health problems in relation to other variables, such as the characteristics and circumstances of the individuals affected" [130] (p. 3).

It has been noted by Davies [146] that "Medicine's ambivalence about accepting domestic violence as a key determinant of health is amply highlighted by the absence in our current ICD of any code for domestic violence" (p. 492). That DSM-5 and ICD-10 has not been forthcoming in clearly naming and linking family violence with Mental Disorders perhaps explains, in part, why mental health practitioners also seem reluctant to assess for and acknowledging the impacts of family violence. It can be confronting to think about how to address the legal, statutory, emotional and safety aspects of addressing family violence [147,148]. Yet more challenging in this work is when infants and very young children are involved. Even those working directly in family violence specific services find it difficult to acknowledge and address the impacts of family violence on children in the early years [49,149]. However, CAMHS is in a powerful position to not only champion the importance of the early identification of family violence, particularly in infancy [43,150–153], but to offer a therapeutic contribution to lives of the families they serve [151,154–160]. Furthermore, CAMHS has much to offer in how the prevalence and complexities of violence within families is thought about from a mental health perspective [49,161–165].

Not every relational stressor may contribute to mental health difficulties in infancy, childhood, adolescence and beyond. Nevertheless, a stressor as prevalent as family violence is alarming. Part of the role of the CAMHS clinician is to assess for and understand how such stressors impact the subjective and psychological experience of the infant, child or adolescent. Speaking plainly about family violence through clarifying terminology, thinking about, responding to and providing intervention and training programs to address the impacts of family violence, CAMHS, as well as adult mental health may do more than provide early intervention and prevention. This may help make sense of and integrate intersectoral responses where children's and "women's experiences of depression, post-traumatic stress, and self-harm can be understood as 'symptoms' or the effects of living with violence and abuse. Domestic violence is not just one of many problems, but an issue that requires addressing as a primary concern" [166] (p.223).

3.1. Identifying and Responding to Family Violence as a Serious Mental Health Issue

Some twenty years ago calls were made by a group of prominent psychiatrists for the DMS-IV to recognise and create a new classification of relational disorders [167]. They argued that there are some problems that cannot be "understood or described by giving a diagnosis to only one individual" (p. 926) and where violence is present that "violence itself is sufficient to diagnose severe couple dysfunction" [167] (p. 928). Essentially, this group believed that the DSM failed to consider that couples as well as families (which includes children) experience severe dysfunction and believed that "family violence involving child or elder abuse, have been omitted from the DSM-IV" [167] (p. 926). A decade ago the Secretary General of the United Nations commissioned the "World Report on Violence Against Children" [168]. This report unequivocally identified the need for a strategic response to "break down the silence in which most children endure episodes of physical, psychological or sexual violence at home" (p. 81). This was in order to recognise that "children who have experienced family violence have a wide range of treatment needs" [168] (p. 84). More recently there have been calls for the upcoming ICD-11 to screen for intimate violence, although these are limited to partner violence [146,169]. The inclusion of 'field tested' diagnostic criteria related to intimate partner violence, Heyman, Slep and Foran [169] argue, could be anticipated to have "even wider and deeper influence in healthcare globally" (p. 78) although they admit "there is no assurance that these, or any other criteria, will be included in ICD-11" (p. 73).

That the DC:0-5 created a new category of Relationship Disorders in 2016 has recognised in part, what the "Committee on the Family" called for in 1995. This is an acknowledgement that "certain problems are relational by their very nature and simply cannot be understood or described by giving a diagnosis to only one individual" [167] (p. 928). This is in contrast to the DSM-5 and ICD-10's continued implication that psychopathology exists within the individual. The DC:0-5 identifies caregiving relationships as central to understanding the infant and young child. Axis II within the DC:0-5 is embedded within a framework which considers the caregiving and relational context as vital to understand in the assessment of infant and young children's development and functioning. Despite this, references to domestic violence were concentrated in the Psychosocial and Environmental Stressor Checklist. Again, omission fails to direct clinicians and practitioners to recognise family violence as a serious risk factor, impinging on the development of good mental health for infants, children and adolescents.

The DC:0-5 sits domestic violence within a checklist which measures a number of co-occurring stresses as more "predictive of subsequent maladaptation than any specific stressors" [7] (p. 153).

Domestic violence is cited as an example of an enduring psychosocial stressor, its impacts understood to be heightened or mitigated by the developmental level of the infant or child, the severity of the violence and the protective buffers offered by the caregivers within that environment "to help the infant/young child understand and cope with the stressor" [7] (p. 153). Including domestic violence as simply one of multiple, possible stressors to impinge on the young child's development does not sufficiently alert CAMHS to the complex, often hidden and urgent imperatives which need to be responded to when an infant or young child is living with family violence, nor how to effectively respond to and treat this high-risk issue.

Community, justice based services and community health services have led the way in developing specific treatment responses for children and women impacted by family violence [41,155,170–175]. Similarly, community based men's behaviour treatment programs, developed to address men's violence, have existed for decades [176–180]. Interventions focusing on reparative work with children and their fathers after family violence is relatively newer territory [158,181] as is any concentrated treatment approach for women who perpetrate violence within intimate relationships, or support programs for men who are victims of family violence [21,22,136,182–184]. Considerably fewer treatment programs to address the impacts of family violence have been developed within CAMHS settings, or within mental health generally, but where they have, there is a strong focus on infants [151,156–158,162,185,186]. Community based approaches to working with family violence have tended to eschew a recognition of mental health issues or approaches [166,178,187]. Given the high correlation between mental health issues and family violence, there would be much to be gained by bringing these differing services together (including the judicial system) to build new, stronger and more efficacious treatment responses to family violence.

3.2. Limitations

It is impossible to capture every conceivable relational stressor that may contribute to mental health difficulties in infancy, childhood, adolescence and beyond. There are other, high prevalence and significant stressors where it could equally be argued greater recognition and acknowledgement is needed within the pages of the DSM-5 and ICD-10. It cannot be definitively argued that family violence has more impact necessarily than another stressor such as early neglect, and/or sexual abuse, both of which carry monumentally damaging risk factors [188–193]. The high correlation between one form of adversity and others (for example child abuse, homelessness etc., and family violence) also adds additional complexities not covered in this paper [44,99,194]. The sheer size of these classification manuals, the diversity of issues needing to be covered and the complexities in the uniformity of definitions leaves it open to criticism's such as have been covered in this paper [9,167,169]. Furthermore, it needs to be noted that the sheer work involved in tabulating the results of the vast number of working groups that contribute to each diagnosis and the lengthy time line between the publication of each version of the DSM hinders its ability to quickly incorporate new research methods such as has "emerged through remarkable advances in new technologies and substantive knowledge in neuroscience" [195] (p. 28).

4. Conclusions

The APA declares that DSM-5 (online version) is "the most comprehensive, current, and critical resource for clinical practice available to today's mental health clinicians and researchers of all orientations. DSM-5 is used by health professionals, social workers, and forensic and legal specialists to diagnose and classify mental disorders" [196]. The ICD-10 claims it "is the foundation for the identification of health trends and statistics globally" [6]. DC:0-5 states that it is not in competition with the ICD-10 and DSM-5 but that "current versions of the latter do not adequately cover syndromes in the earliest postnatal years—syndromes that clinicians encounter and may require urgent attention and preventative interventions" [7] (p. ii). However, all three classification manuals omit clear and consistent references to family violence as a serious risk factor in the development of mental health issues for infants, children, adolescents and adults. Given the extraordinarily high rates of family violence across the world, and the ample evidence of the deleterious impacts of family violence on not just adults, and in particular women [34,118,121,122,132,134,135,197], but on infants, children and adolescents [42,43,45,95,99,100,198–200], there is an urgent need for family violence to be appropriately acknowledged and clearly recognised within the pages of DSM and ICD classifications. DSM-5 and ICD-10. These three key international adult and child mental disorder classification manuals are long overdue in needing to acknowledge family violence as a serious risk factor in the development of mental health symptoms and disorders for infants, children and adolescents. Families seeking help from CAMHS cannot wait, however, for such classification manuals to catch up. Infants, children and adolescents and their families affected by family violence need CAMHS to act now.

Acknowledgments: No funds nor grants were received in support of this work. No funds were received for covering the costs to publish in open access, the fee was waived by the publisher. The authors would like to thank Julie Stone and Sanjay Patel for their feedback on the final draft this paper.

Conflicts of Interest: The authors declare no conflict of interest.

References

1. World Health Organization (WHO). *The World Health Report 2005: Make Every Mother and Child Count*; WHO: Lyon, France, 2005.
2. World Health Organization (WHO). *Global and Regional Estimates of Violence against Women*; WHO: Geneva, Switzerland, 2013.
3. World Health Organization (WHO). *Global Status Report on Violence Prevention 2014*; WHO: Luxembourg, 2014.
4. Carpenter, G.L.; Stacks, A.M. Developmental effects of exposure to intimate partner violence in early childhood: A review of the literature. *Child. Youth Serv. Rev.* **2009**, *31*, 831–839. [CrossRef]
5. American Psychiatric Association (APA). *Diagnostic and Statistical Manual of Mental Disorders (DSM-5)*; APA: St. Louis, MI, USA, 2013.
6. World Health Organization (WHO). *International Statistical Classification of Diseases and Related Health Problems*; WHO: Geneva, Switzerland, 2016.
7. Zero-to-Three. *Diagnostic Classification of Mental Health and Developmental Disorders of Infancy and Early Childhood (DC:0–5)*; ZERO TO THREE: Washington, DC, USA, 2016.
8. Tolan, P.; Gorman-Smith, D.; Henry, D. Family Violence. *Annu. Rev. Psychol.* **2006**, *57*, 557–583. [CrossRef] [PubMed]
9. Kelly, J.B.; Johnson, M.P. Differentiation among types of intimate partner violence: Research update and implications for interventions. *Fam. Court Rev.* **2008**, *46*, 476–499. [CrossRef]
10. European Union Agency for Fundamental Rights. *Violence against Women: An EU-Wide Survey*; FRA: Vienna, Austria, 2014.
11. Phillips, J.; Vandenbroek, P. *Domestic, Family and Sexual Violence in Australia: An Overview of the Issues*; Parliament of Australia: Canberra, Australia, 2014.
12. Breiding, M.J.; Breiding, M.J.; Basile, K.C.; Smith, S.G.; Black, M.C.; Mahendra, R. *Intimate Partner Violence Surveillance: Uniform Definitions and Recommended Data Elements*; National Center for Injury Prevention and Control: Atlanta, GA, USA, 2015.
13. Hines, D.A.; Malley-Morrison, K.; Dutton, L.B. *Family Violence in the United States: Defining, Understanding, and Combating Abuse*, 2nd ed.; Sage Publications: Thousand Oaks, CA, USA, 2013.
14. Yoshihama, M.; Dabby, C. *Facts & Stats Report: Domestic Violence in Asian & Pacific Islander Homes*; Asian & Pacific Islander Institute on Domestic Violence: San Francisco, CA, USA, 2015.
15. Smith, S.G.; Chen, J.; Basile, K.C.; Gilbert, L.K.; Merrick, M.T.; Patel, N.; Walling, M.; Jain, A. *The National Intimate Partner and Sexual Violence Survey (NISVS): 2010–2012 State Report*; National Center for Injury Prevention and Control: Atlanta, GA, USA, 2017.
16. Wahab, S.; Olson, L. Intimate partner violence and sexual assault in Native American communities. *Trauma Violence Abuse* **2004**, *5*, 353–366. [CrossRef] [PubMed]
17. World Health Organization (WHO). *Violence Prevention: The Evidence*; WHO: Geneva, Switzerland, 2009.

18. Alhabib, S.; Nur, U.; Jones, R. Domestic violence against women: Systematic review of prevalence studies. *J. Fam. Violence* **2010**, *25*, 369–382. [CrossRef]

19. Hussain, S.; Usman, M.; Sabir, M.; Zakar, R.; Usmen, A. Prevalence of Spousal Violence and Associated Risk Factors: Facts from pakistan demographics and health survey 2012–2013. *J. Fam. Violence* **2017**, *32*, 711–719. [CrossRef]

20. UN-WOMEN. *Annual Report*; United Nations: New York, NY, USA, 2015–2016.

21. Frieze, I.H. Female violence against intimate partners: An introduction. *Psychol. Women Q.* **2005**, *29*, 229–237. [CrossRef]

22. Douglas, E.; Hines, D. The helpseeking experiences of men who sustain intimate partner violence: An overlooked population and implications for practice. *J. Fam. Violence* **2011**, *26*, 473–485. [CrossRef] [PubMed]

23. Richardson, D.S. The myth of female passivity: Thirty years of revelations about female aggression. *Psychol. Women Q.* **2005**, *29*, 238–247. [CrossRef]

24. Balsam, K.F.; Szymanski, D.M. Relationship quality and domestic violence in women's same-sex relationships: The role of minority stress. *Psychol. Women Q.* **2005**, *29*, 258–269. [CrossRef]

25. Owen, S.S.; Burke, T.W. An exploration of prevalence of domestic violence in same-sex relationships. *Psychol. Rep.* **2004**, *95*, 129–132. [CrossRef] [PubMed]

26. Stanley, J.L.; Bartholomew, K.; Taylor, T.; Oram, D.; Landolt, M. Intimate violence in male same-sex relationships. *J. Fam. Violence* **2006**, *21*, 31–41. [CrossRef]

27. Hellemans, S. Prevalence and impact of intimate partner violence (IPV) among an ethnic minority population. *J. Interpers. Violence* **2014**, *30*, 3389–3481. [CrossRef] [PubMed]

28. Koenig, M.A.; Loeys, T.; Buysse, A.; De Smet, O. Individual and contextual determinants of domestic violence in North India. *Am. J. Public Health* **2006**, *96*, 132–138. [CrossRef] [PubMed]

29. Finkelhor, D.; Turner, H.A.; Shattuck, A.; Hamby, S.L. Prevalence of childhood exposure to violence, crime, and abuse: Results from the national survey of children's exposure to violence. *JAMA Pediatr.* **2015**, *169*, 746–754. [CrossRef] [PubMed]

30. Hamby, S.; Finkelhor, D.; Turner, H.; Ormrod, R. The overlap of witnessing partner violence with child maltreatment and other victimizations in a nationally representative survey of youth. *Child Abuse Negl.* **2010**, *34*, 734–741. [CrossRef] [PubMed]

31. Jewkes, R. Intimate partner violence: Causes and prevention. *The Lancet* **2002**, *359*, 1423–1429. [CrossRef]

32. Buckner, J.C.; Bassuk, E.L.; Zima, B.T. Mental health issues affecting homeless women: Implications for intervention. *Am. J. Orthopsychiatry* **1993**, *63*, 385–399. [CrossRef] [PubMed]

33. Wenzel, S.L.; Leake, B.D.; Gelberg, L. Risk factors for major violence among homeless women. *J. Interpers. Violence* **2001**, *16*, 739–752. [CrossRef]

34. Easton, C.J.; Swan, S.; Sinha, R. Prevalence of family violence in clients entering substance abuse treatment. *J. Subst. Abuse Treat.* **2000**, *18*, 23–28. [CrossRef]

35. National Council to Reduce Violence against Women and their Children (NCRVWC). *The Cost of Violence against Women and Their Children*; NCRVWC: Canberra, Australia, 2009.

36. Coy, M.; Kelly, L. *Islands in the Stream: An Evaluation of Four London Independent Domestic Violence Advocacy Schemes*; London Metropolitan University: London, UK, 2011.

37. ZHang, T.; Hoddenbagh, J.; McDonald, S.; Scrim, K. *An Estimation of the Economic Impact of Spousal Violence in Canada, 2009*; Department of Justice: Vancouver, BC, Canada, 2012.

38. Day, T.; McKenna, K.; Bowlus, A. *The Economic Costs of Violence against Women: An Evaluation of the Literature*; The University of Western Ontario: London, ON, Canada, 2005.

39. Fang, X.M.; Fry, D.A.; Ji, K.; Finkelhor, D.; Chen, J.; Lannene, P.; Dunne, M.P. The burden of child maltreatment in China: A systematic review. *Bull. World Health Organ.* **2015**, *93*, 176C–185C. [CrossRef] [PubMed]

40. Bosquet Enlow, M.; Egeland, B.; Blood, E.A.; Wright, R.O.; Wright, R.J. Interpersonal trauma exposure and cognitive development in children to age 8 years: A longitudinal study. *J. Epidemiol. Community Health* **2012**, *66*, 1005–1010. [CrossRef] [PubMed]

41. Campo, M.; Kaspiew, R.; Moore, S.; Tayton, S. *Children Affected by Domestic and Family Violence: A Review of Domestic and Family Violence Prevention, Early Intervention and Response Services*; Australian Institute of Family Studies: Melbourne, Australia, 2014.

42. Levendosky, A.A.; Bogat, G.A.; Martinez-Torteya, C. PTSD symptoms in young children exposed to intimate partner violence. *Violence Women* **2013**, *19*, 187–201. [CrossRef] [PubMed]
43. Lieberman, A.F.; Chu, A.; Van Horn, P.; Harris, W.W. Trauma in early childhood: Empirical evidence and clinical implications. *Dev. Psychopathol.* **2011**, *23*, 397–410. [CrossRef] [PubMed]
44. Osofsky, J.D. Prevalence of children's exposure to domestic violence and child maltreatment: Implications for prevention and intervention. *Clin. Child Fam. Psychol. Rev.* **2003**, *6*, 161–170. [CrossRef] [PubMed]
45. Perry, B.D. Incubated in terror: Neurodevelopmental factors in the 'cycle of violence'. In *Children in a Violent Society*; Osofsky, J.D., Ed.; The Guilford Press: New York, NY, USA, 1997; pp. 124–149.
46. Davies, C.; Evans, S.E.; DiLillo, D. Exposure to domestic violence: A meta-analysis of child and adolescent outcomes. *Aggress. Violent Behav.* **2008**, *13*, 131–140.
47. Hamby, S.L.; Finkelhor, D.; Turner, H.; Ormrod, R. Children's exposure to intimate partner violence and other family violence: Nationally representative rates among US youth. In *OJJDP Juvenile Justice Bulletin—NCJ 232272*; U.S. Department of Justice: Washington, DC, USA, 2011; pp. 1–12.
48. Mertin, P.; Mohr, P.B. Incidence and correlates of posttrauma symptoms in children from backgrounds of domestic violence. *Violence Vict.* **2002**, *17*, 555–567. [CrossRef] [PubMed]
49. Bunston, W. *Helping Babies and Children (0–6) to Heal after Family Violence: A Practical Guide to Infant- and Child-Led Practice*; Jessica Kingsley Publishers: London, UK, 2017.
50. Garcia-Moreno, C.; Heise, L.; Jansen, H.A.F.M.; Ellsberg, E.; Watts, C. Violence against women. *Science* **2005**, *310*, 1282–1283. [CrossRef] [PubMed]
51. Menezes-Cooper, T. Domestic violence and pregnancy: A literature review. *Int. J. Childbirth Educ.* **2013**, *28*, 30–33.
52. Asling-Monemi, K.; Pena, R.; Ellsberg, M.C.; Persson, L.A. Violence against women increases the risk of infant and child mortality: A case—Referent study in Nicaragua. *Bull. World Health Organ.* **2003**, *81*, 10–18. [PubMed]
53. Bailey, B.A. Partner violence during pregnancy: Prevalence, effects, screening, and management. *Int. J. Women's Health* **2010**, *2*, 183–197. [CrossRef]
54. Coker, A.L.; Sanderson, M.; Dong, B. Partner violence during pregnancy and risk of adverse pregnancy outcomes. *Paediatr. Perinat. Epidemiol.* **2004**, *18*, 260–269. [CrossRef] [PubMed]
55. Jasinski, J.L. Pregnancy and domestic violence: A review of the literature. *Trauma Violence Abuse* **2004**, *5*, 47–64. [CrossRef] [PubMed]
56. Menon, S. Unfinished Lives: The Effect of Domestic Violence on Neonatal and Infant Mortality. 2014. Available online: http://hdl.handle.net/10419/126472 (accessed on 30 July 2015).
57. Quinlivan, J.A.; Evans, S.F. A prospective cohort study of the impact of domestic violence on young teenage pregnancy outcomes. *J. Pediatr. Adolesc. Gynecol.* **2001**, *14*, 17–23. [CrossRef]
58. Taft, A.J.; Watson, L.F.; Lee, C. Violence against young Australian women and association with reproductive events: A cross-sectional analysis of a national population sample. *Aust. N. Z. J. Public Health* **2004**, *28*, 324–329. [CrossRef] [PubMed]
59. Hillis, S.D.; Anda, R.F.; Dube, S.R.; Felitti, V.J.; Marchbanks, P.A.; Marks, J.S. The association between adverse childhood experiences and adolescent pregnancy, long-term psychosocial consequences, and fetal death. *Pediatrics* **2004**, *113*, 320–327. [CrossRef] [PubMed]
60. Lam, W.K.K.; Fals-Stewart, W.; Kelley, M. The timeline followback interview to assess children's exposure to partner violence: Reliability and validity. *J. Fam. Violence* **2009**, *24*, 133–143. [CrossRef]
61. Australian Bureau of Statistics (ABS). *Personal Safety Survey Australia 2012*; ABS: Canberra, Australia, 2012.
62. Meaney, M.J. Epigenetics and the biological definition of gene × environment interactions. *Child Dev.* **2010**, *81*, 41–79. [CrossRef] [PubMed]
63. Shonkoff, J.P.; Phillips, D.A. *From Neurons to Neighborhoods: The Science of Early Childhood Development*; National Academy Press: Washington, DC, USA, 2000.
64. Siegel, D.J. Interpersonal neurobiology as a lens into the development of wellbeing and reslience. *Child. Aust.* **2015**, *40*, 160–164. [CrossRef]
65. Johnson, K. Maternal-infant bonding: A review of literature. *Int. J. Childbirth Educ.* **2013**, *28*, 17–22.
66. Luoma, I.; Kaukonen, P.; Mantymaa, M.; Puura, K.; Tamminen, T.; Salmelin, R. A longitudinal study of maternal depressive symptoms, negative expectations and perceptions of child problems. *Child Psychiatry Hum. Dev.* **2004**, *35*, 37–53. [CrossRef] [PubMed]

67. Clark, C.L.; St. John, N.; Pasca, A.M.; Hyde, S.A.; Hornbeak, K.; Abramova, M.; Feldman, H.; Parker, K.J.; Penn, A.A. Neonatal CSF oxytocin levels are associated with parent report of infant soothability and sociability. *Psychoneuroendocrinology* **2013**, *38*, 1208–1212. [CrossRef] [PubMed]

68. Weatherston, D.; Fitzgerald, H.E. Role of Parenting in the Development of the Infants Interpersonal Abilities. In *Parenthood and Mental Health*; Tyano, S., Keren, M., Herrman, H., Cox, J., Eds.; Wiley-Blackwell: Oxford, UK, 2010; pp. 181–191.

69. Swain, J.E.; Lorberbaum, J.P.; Kose, S.; Strathearn, L. Brain basis of early parent—Infant interactions: Psychology, physiology, and in vivo functional neuroimaging studies. *J. Child Psychol. Psychiatry* **2007**, *48*, 262–287. [CrossRef] [PubMed]

70. Beijers, R.; Risken-Walraven, M.J.; de Weerth, C. Cortisol regulation in 12-month-old human infants: Associations with the infants' early history of breastfeeding and co-sleeping. *Stress* **2013**, *16*, 267–277. [CrossRef] [PubMed]

71. Madigan, S.; Atkinson, L.; Laurin, K.; Benoit, D. Attachment and internalizing behavior in early childhood: A meta-analysis. *Dev. Psychol.* **2013**, *49*, 672–689. [CrossRef] [PubMed]

72. Raby, K.L.; Cicchetti, D.; Carlson, E.A.; Cutuli, J.J.; Englund, M.M.; Egeland, B. Genetic and caregiving-based contributions to infant attachment: Unique associations with distress reactivity and attachment security. *Psychol. Sci.* **2012**, *23*, 1016–1023. [CrossRef] [PubMed]

73. Schore, J.R.; Schore, A.N. Modern attachment theory: The central role of affect regulation in development and treatment. *Clin. Soc. Work J.* **2008**, *36*, 9–20. [CrossRef]

74. Siegel, D.J. *Developing Mind: How Relationships and the Brain Interact to Shape Who We Are*, 2nd ed.; Guilford Press: New York, NY, USA, 2012.

75. Porges, S.W. Making the world safe for our children: Down-regulating defence and up-regulating social engagement to 'optimise' the human experience. *Child. Aust.* **2015**, *40*, 114–123. [CrossRef]

76. Schwerdtfeger, K.L.; Goff, B.S.N. Intergenerational transmission of trauma: Exploring mother-infant prenatal attachment. *J. Trauma. Stress* **2007**, *20*, 39–51. [CrossRef] [PubMed]

77. Huth-Bocks, A.C.; Levendosky, A.A.; Theran, S.A.; Bogat, G.A. The impact of domestic violence on mothers' prenatal representations of their infants. *Infant Ment. Health J.* **2004**, *25*, 79–98. [CrossRef]

78. Huth-Bocks, A.C.; Levendosky, A.A.; Bogat, G.A.; Von Eye, A. The impact of maternal characteristics and contextual variables on infant-mother attachment. *Child Dev.* **2004**, *75*, 480–496. [CrossRef] [PubMed]

79. Huth-Bocks, A.C.; Theran, S.A.; Levendosky, A.A.; Bogat, G.A. A social-contextual understanding of concordance and discordance between maternal prenatal representations of the infant and infant-mother attachment. *Infant Ment. Health J.* **2011**, *32*, 405–426. [CrossRef] [PubMed]

80. Levendosky, A.A.; Bogat, A.G.; Huth-Bocks, A.C. The influence of domestic violence on the development of the attachment relationship between mother and young child. *Psychoanal. Psychol.* **2011**, *28*, 512–527. [CrossRef]

81. Levendosky, A.A.; Lannert, B.; Yalch, M. The effects of intimate partner violence on women and child survivors: An attachment perspective. *Psychodyn. Psychiatry* **2012**, *40*, 397–433. [CrossRef] [PubMed]

82. De Zulueta, F. Understanding the evolution of psychopathology and violence. *Crim. Behav. Ment. Health* **2001**, *11*, S17–S22. [CrossRef]

83. Feldman, S.; Downey, G. Rejection sensitivity as a mediator of the impact of childhood exposure to family violence on adult attachment behavior. *Dev. Psychopathol.* **2008**, *6*, 231–247. [CrossRef] [PubMed]

84. Kuijpers, K.; van der Knaap, L.; Winkel, F. Risk of revictimization of intimate partner violence: The role of attachment, anger and violent behavior of the victim. *J. Fam. Violence* **2012**, *27*, 33–44. [CrossRef] [PubMed]

85. Bowlby, J. Violence in the family as a disorder of the attachment and caregiving systems. *Am. J. Psychoanal.* **1984**, *44*, 9–27. [CrossRef] [PubMed]

86. Schore, A.N. Back to basics attachment, affect regulation, and the developing right brain: Linking developmental neuroscience to pediatrics. *Pediatr. Rev.* **2005**, *26*, 204–217. [CrossRef] [PubMed]

87. Fonagy, P.; Luyten, P.; Strathearn, L. Borderline personality disorder, mentalization, and the neurobiology of attachment. *Infant Ment. Health J.* **2011**, *32*, 47–69. [CrossRef] [PubMed]

88. Hesse, E.; Main, M. Disorganized infant, child, and adult attachment: Collapse in behavioral and attentional strategies. *J. Am. Psychoanal. Assoc.* **2000**, *48*, 1097–1127. [CrossRef] [PubMed]

89. Hesse, E.; Main, M. Frightened, threatening, and dissociative parental behavior in low-risk samples: Description, discussion, and interpretations. *Dev. Psychopathol.* **2006**, *18*, 309–343. [CrossRef] [PubMed]

90. Samuelson, K.W.; Krueger, C.E.; Wilson, C. Relationships between maternal emotion regulation, parenting, and children's executive functioning in families exposed to intimate partner violence. *J. Interpers. Violence* **2012**, *27*, 3532–3550. [CrossRef] [PubMed]

91. Ahlfs-Dunn, S.M.; Huth-Bocks, A.C. Intimate partner violence and infant socioemotional development: The moderating effects of maternal trauma symptoms. *Infant Ment. Health J.* **2014**, *35*, 322–335. [CrossRef] [PubMed]

92. Briggs-Gowan, M.J.; Carter, A.S.; Ford, J.D. Parsing the effects violence exposure in early childhood: Modeling developmental pathways. *J. Pediatr. Psychol.* **2012**, *37*, 11–22. [CrossRef] [PubMed]

93. Graham-Bermann, S.; Howell, K.H.; Miller, L.E.; Kwek, J.; Lilly, M.M. Traumatic events and maternal education as predictors of verbal ability for preschool children exposed to intimate partner violence (IPV). *J. Fam. Violence* **2010**, *25*, 383–392. [CrossRef]

94. Holt, S.; Buckley, H.; Whelan, S. The impact of exposure to domestic violence on children and young people: A review of the literature. *Child Abuse Negl.* **2008**, *32*, 797–810. [CrossRef] [PubMed]

95. Schechter, D.S.; Willheim, E. The effects of violent experiences on infants and young children. In *Handbook of Infant Mental Health*; Zeanah, C.H., Ed.; The Guilford Press: New York, NY, USA, 2009; pp. 197–213.

96. Kitzmann, K.M.; Gaylord, N.K.; Holt, A.R.; Kenny, E.D. Child witnesses to domestic violence: A meta-analytic review. *J. Consult. Clin. Psychol.* **2003**, *71*, 339–352. [CrossRef] [PubMed]

97. Margolin, G.; Vickerman, K.A. Posttraumatic stress in children and adolescents exposed to family violence: I. Overview and issues. *Profess. Psychol. Res. Pract.* **2007**, *38*, 613. [CrossRef] [PubMed]

98. Pelcovitz, D.; Kaplan, S.J.; DeRosa, R.R.; Mandel, F.S.; Salzinger, S. Psychiatric disorders in adolescents exposed to domestic violence and physical abuse. *Am. J. Orthopsychiatry* **2000**, *70*, 360–369. [CrossRef] [PubMed]

99. Moylan, C.A.; Herrenkohl, T.I.; Sousa, C.; Tajima, E.A.; Herrenkohl, R.C.; Russo, M.J. The effects of child abuse and exposure to domestic violence on adolescent internalizing and externalizing behavior problems. *J. Fam. Violence* **2010**, *25*, 53–63. [CrossRef] [PubMed]

100. Sternberg, K.J.; Lamb, M.E.; Gutermana, E.; Abbotta, C.B. Effects of early and later family violence on children's behavior problems and depression: A longitudinal, multi-informant perspective. *Child Abuse Negl.* **2006**, *30*, 283–306. [CrossRef] [PubMed]

101. Schore, A.N. *Affect Regulation and the Origin of the Self: The Neurobiology of Emotional Development*; Routledge: New York, NY, USA, 2016.

102. Tronick, E.Z. *The Neurobehavioral and Social-Emotional Development of Infants and Children*; W.W. Norton & Company: New York, NY, USA, 2007.

103. Teicher, M.H.; Andersen, S.L.; Polcari, A.; Anderson, C.M.; Navalta, C.P.; Kim, D.M. The neurobiological consequences of early stress and childhood maltreatment. *Neurosci. Biobehav. Rev.* **2003**, *27*, 33–44. [CrossRef]

104. Cirulli, F.; Berry, A.; Alleva, E. Early disruption of the mother–infant relationship: Effects on brain plasticity and implications for psychopathology. *Neurosci. Biobehav. Rev.* **2003**, *27*, 73–82. [CrossRef]

105. Smith, S.M.; Vale, W.W. The role of the hypothalamic-pituitary-adrenal axis in neuroendocrine responses to stress. *Dialogues Clin. Neurosci.* **2006**, *8*, 383–395. [PubMed]

106. Murri, M.B.; Prestia, D.; Mondelli, V.; Pariante, C.; Patti, S.; Olivieri, B.; Arzani, C.; Masotti, M.; Respino, M.; Antonioli, M.; et al. The HPA axis in bipolar disorder: Systematic review and meta-analysis. *Psychoneuroendocrinology* **2016**, *63*, 327–342. [CrossRef] [PubMed]

107. Carrion, V.; Wong, S.; Kletter, H. Update on neuroimaging and cognitive functioning in maltreatment-related pediatric PTSD: Treatment implications. *J. Fam. Violence* **2013**, *28*, 53–61. [CrossRef]

108. Schechter, D.S.; Hao, X.; Duan, Y.; Marsh, R.; Yu, S.; Wang, Z.; Kangarlu, A.; Gunter, B.; Murphy, D.; McCaw, J.E.; et al. An fMRI study of the brain responses of traumatized mothers to viewing their toddlers during separation and play. *Soc. Cognit. Affect. Neurosci.* **2012**, *7*, 969–979. [CrossRef] [PubMed]

109. Schore, A.N. *Affect Dysregulation and Disorders of the Self*; W.W. Norton & Company: New York, NY, USA, 2003.

110. Graham, A.M.; Fisher, P.A.; Pfeifer, J.H. What sleeping babies hear: A functional MRI study of interparental conflict and infants' emotion processing. *Psychol. Sci.* **2013**, *24*, 782–789. [CrossRef] [PubMed]

111. Rifkin-Graboi, A.; Borelli, J.L.; Enlow, M.B. Neurobiology of stress in infancy. In *Handbook of Infant Mental Health*; Zeanah, C.H., Ed.; The Guilford Press: New York, NY, USA, 2009; pp. 59–79.

112. Gunnar, M.; Quevedo, K. The neurobiology of stress and development. *Annu. Rev. Psychol.* **2007**, *58*, 145–173. [CrossRef] [PubMed]

113. Van der Kolk, B. *The Body Keeps the Score: Brain, Mind, and Body in the Healing of Trauma*; Penguin: London, UK, 2014.

114. McCarron, R.M. The DSM-5 and the art of medicine: Certainly uncertain. *Ann. Intern. Med.* **2013**, *159*, 360–361. [CrossRef] [PubMed]

115. Rosenberg, S.D.; Lu, W.; Mueser, K.T.; Jankowski, M.K.; Cournos, F. Correlates of adverse childhood events among adults with schizophrenia spectrum disorders. *Psychiatr. Serv.* **2007**, *58*, 245–253. [CrossRef] [PubMed]

116. Walsh, E.; Buchanan, A.; Fahy, T. Violence and Schizophrenia: Examining the evidence. *Br. J. Psychiatry* **2002**, *180*, 490–495. [CrossRef] [PubMed]

117. Bebbington, P.E.; Bhugra, D.; Brugha, T.; Singleton, N.; Farrell, M.; Jenk, R.; Meltzer, H. Psychosis, victimisation and childhood disadvantage. *Br. J. Psychiatry* **2004**, *185*, 220–226. [CrossRef] [PubMed]

118. Helfrich, C.A.; Fujiura, G.T.; Rutkowski-Kmitta, V. Mental health disorders and functioning of women in domestic violence shelters. *J. Interpers. Violence* **2008**, *23*, 437–453. [CrossRef] [PubMed]

119. Campbell, R.; Sullivan, C.M.; Davidson, W.S. Women who use domestic violence shelters changes in depression over time. *Psychol. Women Q.* **1995**, *19*, 237–255. [CrossRef]

120. Watlington, C.G.; Murphy, C.M. The roles of religion and spirituality among African American survivors of domestic violence. *J. Clin. Psychol.* **2006**, *62*, 837–857. [CrossRef] [PubMed]

121. Mertin, P.; Mohr, P.B. A follow-up study of posttraumatic stress disorder, anxiety, and depression in Australian victims of domestic violence. *Violence Vict.* **2001**, *16*, 645–654. [PubMed]

122. Tolman, R.M.; Rosen, D. Domestic violence in the lives of women receiving welfare: Mental health, substance dependence, and economic well-being. *Violence Women* **2001**, *7*, 141–158. [CrossRef]

123. Dube, S.R.; Felitti, V.J.; Dong, M.; Chapman, D.P.; Giles, W.H.; Anda, R.F. Childhood abuse, neglect, and household dysfunction and the risk of illicit drug use: The adverse childhood experiences study. *Pediatrics* **2003**, *111*, 564–572. [CrossRef] [PubMed]

124. Fals-Stewart, W.; Kennedy, C. Addressing intimate partner violence in substance-abuse treatment. *J. Subst. Abuse Treat.* **2005**, *29*, 5–17. [CrossRef] [PubMed]

125. Boles, S.M.; Miotto, K. Substance abuse and violence: A review of the literature. *Aggress. Violent Behav.* **2003**, *8*, 155–174. [CrossRef]

126. Sansone, R.A.; Chu, J.; Wiederman, M.W. Domestic violence and borderline personality symptomatology among women in an inpatient psychiatric setting. *Traumatology* **2006**, *12*, 314–319. [CrossRef]

127. Herman, J.L.; Perry, C.; van der Kolk, B.A. Childhood trauma in borderline personality disorder. *Am. J. Psychiatry* **1989**, *146*, 490–495. [PubMed]

128. Hagan, M.J.; Hulette, A.C.; Lieberman, A.F. Symptoms of dissociation in a high-risk sample of young children exposed to interpersonal trauma: Prevalence, correlates, and contributors. *J. Trauma. Stress* **2015**, *28*, 258–261. [CrossRef] [PubMed]

129. Trevillion, K.; Hughes, B.; Feder, G.; Borschmann, R.; Oram, S.; Howard, L. Disclosure of domestic violence in mental health settings: A qualitative meta-synthesis. *Int. Rev. Psychiatry* **2014**, *26*, 430–444. [CrossRef] [PubMed]

130. World Health Organization (WHO). ICD-10 International Statistical Classification of Diseases and Related Health Problems. In *Instruction Manual*; World Health Organization: Lyon, France, 2016.

131. Oram, S.; Trevillion, K.; Feder, G.; Howard, L.M. Prevalence of experiences of domestic violence among psychiatric patients: Systematic review. *Br. J. Psychiatry* **2013**, *202*, 94–99. [CrossRef] [PubMed]

132. Golding, J.M. Intimate partner violence as a risk factor for mental disorders: A meta-analysis. *J. Fam. Violence* **1999**, *14*, 99–132. [CrossRef]

133. Ellsberg, M.; Jansen, H.A.F.M.; Heise, L.; Watts, C.H.; Garcia-Moreno, C. Intimate partner violence and women's physical and mental health in the WHO multi-country study on women's health and domestic violence: An observational study. *The Lancet* **2008**, *371*, 1165–1172. [CrossRef]

134. Coker, A.L.; Davis, K.E.; Arias, I.; Desai, S.; Sanderson, M.; Brandt, H.M.; Smith, P.H. Physical and mental health effects of intimate partner violence for men and women. *Am. J. Prev. Med.* **2002**, *23*, 260–268. [CrossRef]

135. Pico-Alfonso, M.A.; Garcia-Linares, G.M.; Celda-Navarro, N.; Blasco-Ros, C.; Echeburúa, E.; Martinez, M. The impact of physical, psychological, and sexual intimate male partner violence on women's mental health: Depressive symptoms, posttraumatic stress disorder, state anxiety, and suicide. *J. Women's Health* **2006**, *15*, 599–611. [CrossRef] [PubMed]

136. Fanslow, J.L.; Gulliver, P.; Dixon, R.; Ayallo, I. Women's initiation of physical violence against an abusive partner outside of a violent episode. *J. Interpers. Violence* **2014**, *30*, 2659–2682. [CrossRef] [PubMed]
137. Henning, K.; Renauer, B.; Holdford, R. Victim or offender? Heterogeneity among women arrested for intimate partner violence. *J. Fam. Violence* **2006**, *21*, 351–368. [CrossRef]
138. Zero-to-Three. *DC: 0–3R Diagnostic Classification of Mental Health and Developmental Disorders of Infancy and Early Childhood*; Zero-to-Three: Washington, DC, USA, 2005.
139. Perry, B.D. The neurodevelopmental impact of violence in childhood. In *Textbook of Child and Adolescent Forensic Psychiatry*; Schetky, D., Benedek, E.P., Eds.; American Psychiatric Press, Inc.: Washington, DC, USA, 2001; pp. 221–238.
140. Krug, E.G.; Mercy, J.A.; Dahlberg, L.L.; Zwi, A.B. The world report on violence and health. *The Lancet* **2002**, *360*, 1083–1088. [CrossRef]
141. Markowitz, F.E. Attitudes and family violence: Linking intergenerational and cultural theories. *J. Fam. Violence* **2001**, *16*, 205–218. [CrossRef]
142. Beaulaurier, R.L.; Seff, L.R.; Newman, F.L. Barriers to help-seeking for older women who experience intimate partner violence: A descriptive model. *J. Women Aging* **2008**, *20*, 231–248. [CrossRef] [PubMed]
143. Bell, M.E.; Goodman, L.A.; Dutton, M. The dynamics of staying and leaving: Implications for battered women's emotional well-being and experiences of violence at the end of a year. *J. Fam. Violence* **2007**, *22*, 413–428. [CrossRef]
144. Kemp, A.; Green, B.L.; Hovanitz, C.; Rawlings, E.I. Incidence and correlates of posttraumatic stress disorder in battered women: Shelter and community samples. *J. Interpers. Violence* **1995**, *10*, 43–55. [CrossRef]
145. Pajak, C.R.; Ahmad, F.; Jenney, A.; Fisher, P.; Chan, L.M. Survivor's costs of saying no: Exploring the experience of accessing services for intimate partner violence. *J. Interpers. Violence* **2014**, *29*, 2571–2591. [CrossRef] [PubMed]
146. Davies, V. Domestic violence: we need changes in the ICD and at the start of training. *Br. J. Psychiatry* **2011**, *198*, 492–495. [CrossRef] [PubMed]
147. Trevillion, K.; Howard, L.M.; Morgan, C.; Feder, G.; Woodall, A.; Rose, D. The response of mental health services to domestic violence: A qualitative study of service users' and professionals' experiences. *J. Am. Psychiatr. Nurses Assoc.* **2012**, *18*, 326–336. [CrossRef] [PubMed]
148. Rose, D.; Trevillion, K.; Woodall, A.; Morgan, C.; Feder, G.; Howard, L. Barriers and facilitators of disclosures of domestic violence by mental health service users: Qualitative study. *Br. J. Psychiatry* **2010**, *198*, 189–194. [CrossRef] [PubMed]
149. Bunston, W. *How Refuge Provides 'Refuge' to Infants: Exploring How 'Refuge' is Provided to Infants Entering Crisis Accommodation with Their Mothers after Fleeing Family Violence*; La Trobe University: Melbourne, Australia, 2016.
150. Bunston, W. Let's start at the very beginning: The sound of infants, mental health, homelessness and you. *Parity* **2011**, *24*, 37–39.
151. Bunston, W.; Eyre, K.; Carlsson, A.; Pringle, K. Evaluating relational repair work with infants and mothers impacted by family violence. *Aust. N. Z. J. Criminol.* **2016**, *49*, 113–133. [CrossRef]
152. Bunston, W.; Heynatz, A. (Eds.) *Addressing Family Violence Programs: Groupwork Interventions for Infants, Children and Their Parents*; Royal Children's Hospital Mental Health Service: Victoria, Australia, 2006.
153. Lieberman, A.F. Traumatic stress and quality of attachment: Reality and internalization in disorders of infant mental health. *Infant Ment. Health J.* **2004**, *25*, 336–351. [CrossRef]
154. Johnston, J.R. Group interventions for children at-risk from family abuse and exposure to violence. *J. Emot. Abuse* **2003**, *3*, 203–226. [CrossRef]
155. Thompson, E.H.; Trice-Black, S. School-based group interventions for children exposed to domestic violence. *J. Fam. Violence* **2012**, *27*, 233–241. [CrossRef]
156. Lieberman, A.F.; van Horn, P. *Don't Hit My Mommy: A Manual for Child-Parent Psychotherapy with Young Witnesses of Family Violence*; Zero to Three Press: Washington, DC, USA, 2004.
157. Bunston, W. Baby lead the way: Mental health groupwork for infants, children and mothers affected by family violence. *J. Fam. Stud.* **2008**, *14*, 334–341. [CrossRef]
158. Bunston, W. "What about the fathers?" bringing 'Dads on Board™' with their infants and toddlers following violence. *J. Fam. Stud.* **2013**, *19*, 70–79. [CrossRef]

159. Bunston, W. Children exposed to family violence. In *Handbook of Child and Adolescent Therapy*; Haen, C., Aronson, S., Eds.; Routledge: New York, NY, USA, 2017; pp. 404–414.

160. Bunston, W.; Pavlidis, T.; Cartwright, P. Children, family violence and group work: Some do's and don'ts in running therapeutic groups with children affected by family violence. *J. Fam. Violence* **2016**, *31*, 85–94. [CrossRef]

161. Thomson Salo, F. Relating to the infant as subject in the context of family violence. In *The Baby as Subject*; Salo, F.T., Paul, C., Eds.; Stonnington Press: Victoria, Australia, 2007.

162. Lieberman, A.F.; van Horn, P. *Psychotherapy with Infants and Young Children: Repairing the Effects of Stress and Trauma on Early Attachment*; The Guilford Press: New York, NY, USA, 2008.

163. Lieberman, A.F.; van Horn, P. Child-parent psychotherapy. In *Handbook of Infant Mental Health*; Zenah, C.H., Ed.; The Guilford Press: New York, NY, USA, 2009; pp. 439–449.

164. Osofsky, J.D. Perspectives on helping traumatized infants, young children, and their families. *Infant Ment. Health J.* **2009**, *30*, 673–677. [CrossRef] [PubMed]

165. Brinamen, C.F.; Taranta, A.N.; Johnston, K. Expanding early childhood mental health consultation to new venues: Serving infants and young children in domestic violence and homeless shelters. *Infant Ment. Health J.* **2012**, *33*, 283–293. [CrossRef] [PubMed]

166. Humphreys, C.; Thiara, R. Mental health and domestic violence: 'I call it symptoms of abuse'. *Br. J. Soc. Work* **2003**, *33*, 209–226. [CrossRef]

167. Committee on the Family, Group for the Advancement of Psychiatry. A model for the classification and diagnosis of relational disorders. *Psychiatr. Serv.* **1995**, *46*, 926–931.

168. Pinheiro, P.S. *World Report on Violence against Children*; United Nations: Geneva, Switzerland, 2006.

169. Heyman, R.E.; Slep, A.M.S.; Foran, H.M. Enhanced definitions of intimate partner violence for DSM-5 and ICD-11 may promote improved screening and treatment. *Fam. Process* **2015**, *54*, 64–81. [CrossRef] [PubMed]

170. Cunningham, A.J.; Baker, L.L. *Little Eyes, Little Ears: How Violence against a Mother Shapes Children as They Grow*; Centre for Children & Families in the Justice System: London, ON, Canada, 2007.

171. Graham-Bermann, S.A.; Lynch, L.; Banyard, V.; DeVoe, E.R.; Halabu, H. Community-based intervention for children exposed to intimate partner violence: An efficacy trial. *J. Consult. Clin. Psychol.* **2007**, *75*, 199–209. [CrossRef] [PubMed]

172. Keeshin, B.; Oxman, A.; Schindler, S.; Campbell, K.A. A domestic violence shelter parent training program for mothers with young children. *J. Fam. Violence* **2015**, *30*, 461–466. [CrossRef]

173. Stanley, N.; Humphries, C. (Eds.) *Domestic Violence and Protecting Children: New Thinking and Approaches*; Jessica Kingsley Publishers: London, UK, 2015.

174. Groves, B.M. *Children Who See Too Much: Lessons from the Child Witness to Violence Project*; Beacon Press: Boston, MA, USA, 2002.

175. Barron, J. *Kidspeak: Giving Children and Young People a Voice on Domestic Violence*; Women's Aid: Bristol, UK, 2007.

176. Akoensi, T.D.; Koehler, J.A.; Lösel, F.; Humphreys, D.K. Domestic violence perpetrator programs in Europe, Part II: A systematic review of the state of evidence. *Int. J. Offender Ther. Comp. Criminol.* **2013**, *57*, 1206–1225. [CrossRef] [PubMed]

177. Babcock, J.C.; Green, C.E.; Robie, C. Does batterers' treatment work? A meta-analytic review of domestic violence treatment. *Clin. Psychol. Rev.* **2004**, *23*, 1023–1053. [CrossRef] [PubMed]

178. Day, A.; Chung, D.; O'Leary, P.; Carson, E. Programs for men who perpetrate domestic violence: An examination of the issues underlying the effectiveness of intervention programs. *J. Fam. Violence* **2009**, *24*, 203–212. [CrossRef]

179. Maiuro, R.D.; Eberle, J.A. State standards for domestic violence perpetrator treatment: Current status, trends, and recommendations. *Violence Vict.* **2008**, *23*, 133–155. [CrossRef] [PubMed]

180. Sonkin, D.J.; Martin, D.; Walker, L.E. *The Male Batterer: A Treatment Approach*; Springer Publishing Company: New York, NY, USA, 1985; Volume 4.

181. Labarre, M.; Gulliver, P.; Dixon, R.; Ayallo, I. Intervening with fathers in the context of intimate partner violence: An analysis of ten programs and suggestions for a research agenda. *J. Child Custody* **2016**, *13*, 1–29. [CrossRef]

182. Drijber, B.; Reijnders, U.L.; Ceelen, M. Male victims of domestic violence. *J. Fam. Violence* **2013**, *28*, 173–178. [CrossRef]

183. Fanslow, J.L.; Gulliver, P.; Dixon, R.; Ayallo, I. Hitting back: Women's use of physical violence against violent male partners, in the context of a violent episode. *J. Interpers. Violence* **2014**, *30*, 2963–2979. [CrossRef] [PubMed]

184. Milner, J.; Singleton, T. Domestic violence: Solution-focused practice with men and women who are violent. *J. Fam. Ther.* **2008**, *30*, 29–53. [CrossRef]

185. Bunston, W. *Parkas: Parents Accepting Responsibility Kids are Safe*; Mental Health Services for Kids and Youth (MHSKY): Victoria, Australia, 2001.

186. Bunston, W. The Peek a Boo Club: Group work for infants and mothers affected by family violence. *Signal* **2006**, *14*, 1–7.

187. Jewell, L.M.; Wormith, J.S. Variables associated with attrition from domestic violence treatment programs targeting male batterers: A meta-analysis. *Crim. Justice Behav.* **2010**, *37*, 1086–1113. [CrossRef]

188. Afifi, T.O.; Mather, A.; Boman, J.; Fleisher, W.; Enns, M.W.; MacMillan, H.; Sareen, J. Childhood adversity and personality disorders: Results from a nationally representative population-based study. *J. Psychiatr. Res.* **2011**, *45*, 814–822. [CrossRef] [PubMed]

189. Battle, C.L.; Shea, M.T.; Johnson, D.M.; Zlotnick, C.; Zanarini, M.C.; Sanislow, C.A.; Skodol, A.E.; Gunderson, J.G.; Grilo, C.M.; McGlashan, T.H.; et al. Childhood maltreatment associated with adult personality disorders: Findings from the Collaborative Longitudinal Personality Disorders Study. *J. Personal. Disord.* **2004**, *18*, 193–211. [CrossRef]

190. Briere, J.; Elliott, D.M. Prevalence and psychological sequelae of self-reported childhood physical and sexual abuse in a general population sample of men and women. *Child Abuse Negl.* **2003**, *27*, 1205–1222. [CrossRef] [PubMed]

191. Grover, K.E.; Carpenter, L.L.; Price, L.H.; Gagne, G.G.; Mello, A.F.; Mello, M.F.; Tyrka, A.R. The Relationship between Childhood Abuse and Adult Personality Disorder Symptoms. *J. Personal. Disord.* **2007**, *21*, 442–447. [CrossRef] [PubMed]

192. Kendler, K.S.; Bulik, C.M.; Silberg, J.; Hettema, J.M.; Myers, J.; Prescott, C.A. Childhood sexual abuse and adult psychiatric and substance use disorders in women: An epidemiological and cotwin control analysis. *Arch. Gen. Psychiatry* **2000**, *57*, 953–959. [CrossRef] [PubMed]

193. Lobbestael, J.; Arntz, A.; Bernstein, D.P. Disentangling the relationship between different types of childhood maltreatment and personality disorders. *J. Personal. Disord.* **2010**, *24*, 285–295. [CrossRef] [PubMed]

194. Herrenkohl, T.I.; Sousa, C.; Tajima, E.A.; Herrenkohl, R.C.; Moylan, C.A. Intersection of child abuse and children's exposure to domestic violence. *Trauma Violence Abuse* **2008**, *9*, 84–99. [CrossRef] [PubMed]

195. Cuthbert, B.N. The RDoC framework: Facilitating transition from ICD/DSM to dimensional approaches that integrate neuroscience and psychopathology. *World Psychiatry* **2014**, *13*, 28–35. [CrossRef] [PubMed]

196. American Psychiatric Association (APA). *Diagnostic and Statistical Manual of Mental Disorders (DSM-5) Online Version*; APA: St. Louis, MI, USA, 2017.

197. McPherson, M.D.; Delva, J.; Cranford, J.A. A longitudinal investigation of intimate partner violence among mothers with mental illness. *Psychiatr. Serv.* **2007**, *58*, 675–680. [CrossRef] [PubMed]

198. Fantuzzo, J.W.; Fusco, R.A. Children's direct exposure to types of domestic violence crime: A Population-based Investigation. *J. Fam. Violence* **2007**, *22*, 543–552. [CrossRef]

199. Osofsky, J.D. Community outreach for children exposed to violence. *Infant Ment. Health J.* **2004**, *25*, 478–487. [CrossRef]

200. Van der Kolk, B.A. Developmental trauma disorder. *Psychiatr. Ann.* **2005**, *35*, 401–408. [CrossRef]

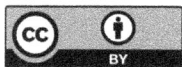

brain
sciences

MDPI

Article

Analysis of Predictive Factors on Minors' Mental Health According to the Spanish National Health Survey

Fernando Fajardo-Bullón [1],* , Irina Rasskin-Gutman [2] , Elena Felipe-Castaño [2],
Eduardo João Ribeiro dos Santos [3] and Benito León-del Barco [2]

[1]   Department of Psychology, Faculty of Education and Psychology, University of Extremadura,
      Badajoz 06006, Spain
[2]   Department of Psychology, Faculty of Teacher Training College, University of Extremadura, Cáceres 10071,
      Spain; irasskin@unex.es (I.R.-G.); efelipe@unex.es (E.F.-C.); bleon@unex.es (B.L.-d.B.)
[3]   Scientific Coordinator R&D Unit Institute of Cognitive Psychology (IPCDHS/FPCE), University of Coimbra,
      Coimbra 3000-115, Portugal; eduardosantos@fpce.uc.pt
*   Correspondence: fernandofajardo@unex.es; Tel.: +34-924-289-300 (ext. 57664)

Received: 5 September 2017; Accepted: 17 October 2017; Published: 21 October 2017

Abstract: Research on minors' mental health is an increasingly developing area. Given the increased prevalence of disorders, it seems necessary to analyze the factors that can affect poor mental health. This study analyzes the influence of occupational class, educational level, age, sex and perceived mental health of Spanish children, which is measured through the Strengths and Difficulties Questionnaire. The sample consists of 3599 minors between 4 and 14 years old, who were interviewed through the Spanish National Health Survey 2011. Our results indicating the significant ($p < 0.05$) relationship between mental health, occupational class (OR 0.533) and minors' health in the last year (OR 0.313) are shown. However, gender (OR 1.187) and educational level of Pre-School Education in relation to Secondary Education (OR 1.174) and Primary Education (OR 0.996) do not generate significant differences. In conclusion, we consider it necessary to design and implement public policies aimed at improving the care system for children who have had poor or regular health in the last year, and whose parents are positioned in the lowest part of the occupational scale.

Keywords: mental health; child welfare; social class; health promotion

1. Introduction

For more than a decade, the problem of mental health in children, with rates of those affected being between 10% and 20%, worldwide, has increased [1,2]. We know that new generations are now more likely to have mental health problems than previous ones, and that inadequate mental health may be linked with suicide cases, which are the second and third causes of teenage mortality, according to several international studies reviewed [3]. If, at the same time, we take into account that 50% of adults' disorders had their onset in adolescence, it seems necessary to perform an analysis of the factors that affect the mental health of minors, not only as a treatment measure, but also with the aim of preventing future disorders [4,5]. In fact, the presence of mental health problems in the parents could be a predictor of mental health problems in children, and therefore this situation would form a cycle where the difficulties could pass from parents to children [6].

Two main difficulties for this analysis are the use of different questionnaires that make difficult to compare the international samples studied, as well as the fact that local studies do not allow the generalization of the results. To overcome these obstacles, the Strengths and Difficulties Questionnaire (SDQ)—parents version [5,7]—has been implemented in this study. This questionnaire has been used with a Spanish population previously [6,8,9], and has demonstrated good qualities for measuring mental health at a national and international level, especially with its scoring at the total scale in difficulties [7,10]. In the present study, we use the same scale as was included in the Spanish National Health Survey (ENSE, 2011–2012) [8,11]. This questionnaire, in its 'parents' version, has proved to be a good tool for the screening of mental disorders in cross-cultural studies in European countries, establishing itself as an international mental health measurement tool [12].

Several reports indicate the need to analyze which variables affect the mental health of minors, and encourage the social sciences to collect data in order to clarify the increase of mental health problems in minors in Western countries [2,10,13–15]. According to previous analyses with Spanish national samples, it seems that the occupational class of parents could be a relevant variable for the mental health of minors [16], with less favored classes predicting worse results in the mental health of minors. As in North America, those with low-income parents associated with low occupational classes had higher levels of depression and anxiety [17], and may even experience feelings of helplessness and inferiority, or behaviors of alcohol abuse [18]. Given the economic crisis in Spain since 2008, it seems necessary to analyze the variables that may affect the mental health of Spanish minors. Therefore, the objective of this study is to analyze the influence of variables such as "occupational class of the parents", "educational level", "sex" and "perceived health"—according to the 2011 Spanish National Health Survey—on the mental health of Spanish children aged between 4 and 14 years old.

2. Materials and Methods

2.1. Participants

The Spanish National Health Survey (ENSE-2011/12) [11] collects health information relative to the resident population in Spain in 21,508 households, these being the main dwellings. The sample size was 26,502 interviews, 21,007 adults (15 and over), and 5495 children (0–14 years), the latter by interviewing their parents/guardians. In this study, we have worked exclusively with the results of the survey related to minors from 4 to 14, and whose responses were obtained by their parents. Therefore, our study is based on a sample of 3599 children. 52.49% male, 17.45% between 4 and 5 years old, 62.24% between 6 and 12 years old, and 20.31% between 13 and 14 years old (Table 1). These data were collected between July 2011 and June 2012. In order to achieve the goals of the survey and provide estimation with a certain degree of reliability (both in national and regional levels), a sample of 24,000 dwellings distributed in 2000 census sections was selected. There were 12 dwellings selected in each census section. To determine the size of the sample, the type of characteristics studied, the information provided by the selected respondents, and the importance of the representativeness of the study of children were taken into account. The sample was distributed among the regions (Spanish Autonomous Communities), assigning one equitable part and another taking into account the proportion of the region size. Sections were selected for each stratum based on the probability proportional to their size. That is to say that the dwellings in each section would have the same probability via random systematic sampling, and the procedure allowed self-weighted samples in each stratum to be obtained. More information regarding this procedure is available from the Ministry of Health, Social Services and Equality.

2.2. Instrument

The instrument used was the SDQ-parent questionnaire [7]. It has been translated into 66 languages and internationally validated [9,19,20]. It is an instrument of excellent quality for the screening of mental health in minors, and its usability, as well as the reliability of the scores, makes it very attractive for research [21,22]. It consists of 5 scales of 5 items each. The total score for difficulties is calculated based on the sum of the first 4 scales (emotional symptoms, behavior problems, hyperactivity, problems with peers), avoiding the sum of the last scale (prosocial), as has been established in the methodology of previous research using the SDQ, including that of Goodman and Goodman, its creators [22]. To facilitate the analysis of mental health, once the answers had been obtained, the score of each minor—that would vary between 0 and 40 points—was divided into two categories: suffering or not suffering from mental health problems, based on whether the total score was greater than or equal to 20 points (suffer) or less than 20 points (not suffering) [9,23]. This variable was contrasted with the complementary sociodemographic information obtained through interview: occupational class, educational level, sex, and perceived health. Six occupational social classes were considered, based on the Spanish adaptation of the British Registrar General classification [24]. The authors grouped them into three social classes for better study: class 1 (combining the most privileged social classes I and II), class 2 (combining the middle classes III and IVa) and class 3 (combining classes less privileged in that register; IVb and V). Additionally, based on the minors' age, three corresponding educational levels were considered: Pre-School Education (children between four and five years old), Primary Education (minors between six and 12 years old) and Compulsory Secondary Education (ESO) (13 and 14 years old). For the perceived health in the last year, three levels were considered: "good or very good", "regular", and "bad or very bad".

2.3. Procedure

The type of sampling used was stratified tri-stage. The information corresponding to the questionnaire for minors was obtained indirectly, facilitated in our case by the mother or the father. The method of collecting information was Computer-Assisted Personal Interviews (CAPI), direct in the case of adults, and the mother/father or guardian. This is to say that, in our study, we have only selected those responses by parents of the minors. This survey was approved by the Committee of Good Practices of the European Statistical System (ETUCE) under the protocol of action of the National Institute of Statistics and Ministry of Health Social Services and Equality developed by ENSE-2011 (Directive 95/46/Parliament and the European Council of 24 October 1995 on the protection of individuals with regard to the processing of personal data and on the free movement of such data).

2.4. Analyitic Approach

Analysis of variance techniques (ANOVA) were used to analyze whether there were significant differences between the total score obtained in the SDQ-parent test and the independent variables or selected factors, such as sex, educational level, occupational class, and perceived health. In order to analyze the association between having or mental health problems or not with respect to the risk factors mentioned above, we used the statistical tools of odds ratio (OR) and relative risks (risk ratio, RR). In this last analysis, we used the occupational social class 3 (less privileged) and Compulsory Secondary Education as comparative control classes. For the regression analysis, 189 subjects with missing or incomplete observations were eliminated. The remaining subjects in the sample were all included.

3. Results

In Table 1, the frequency distribution and percentages of the mean of the scores reached in the SDQ test, 'parent version', can be observed, according to the risk factors chosen.

A priori, there appear to be significant differences in means in the sex factor, the educational level factor, the occupational class factor and among the three categories of the perceived health factor (Table 2).

Through the analysis of a general univariate linear model, the sex factor ($F = 14.372$; $p = 0.000$) and the educational level factor show significant differences ($F = 5.388$, $p = 0.0048$). Scheffé's post hoc tests show that these significant differences exist between Pre-School Education and all other categories (Primary and Secondary Education), and there are no significant differences between the categories Primary Education and Secondary Education. In addition to this, minors who are in Pre-School Education have a higher propensity to suffer mental health problems.

Table 1. Descriptive statistics according to the studied variables.

Variables	N (%)	[a] SDQ's Ratings M (DT)
Sex		
Male	1889 (52.49)	8.78 (5.53)
Female	1710 (47.51)	8.09 (5.43)
Total	3599 (100)	8.45 (5.49)
Education		
Pre-School (4–5 years old)	628 (17.45)	9.08 (5.33)
Primary (6–12 years old)	2240 (62.24)	8.34 (5.49)
Secondary (13–14 years old)	731 (20.31)	8.24 (5.61)
Total	3599 (100)	8.45 (5.49)
Occupational Class		
Class 1	720 (21.11)	7.38 (4.95)
Class 2	1172 (34.37)	8.27 (5.41)
Class 3	1518 (44.52)	9.13 (5.66)
Total	3410 (100)	8.46 (5.47)
Perceived Health		
Good or very good	3367 (93.58)	8.22 (5.31)
Regular	211 (5.86)	11.60 (6.72)
Bad or very bad	20 (0.56)	14.50 (7.30)
Total	3598 (100)	8.45 (5.49)

[a] SDQ = Strengths and Difficulties Questionnaire.

Table 2. Ordinary Least Squares Model.

	Coefficient	DT	t	p
Constant	4.8829	0.5903	8.2705	<0.0001
Sex	−0.7253	0.1826	−3.9714	<0.0001
Occupational Class	0.8356	0.1177	7.0974	<0.0001
Perceived Health	3.3601	0.3283	10.2342	<0.0001
Age	−0.2728	0.0684	−3.9863	<0.0001

R^2 = 0.055 (5.5%); $F(3,3404)$ = 40.007; Value $p < 0.001$.

As far as the occupational class is concerned, there were significant differences between the means of their categories ($F = 26.391$, $p = 0.000$) and there were significant differences among the three occupational level classes in Scheffé's post hoc tests.

Finally, in relation to perceived health in the last year, significant differences were obtained between the means of perceived health levels ($F = 51.172$, $p = 0.000$). Furthermore, through Scheffé's post hoc tests, different means were obtained in the three levels, with minors who presented poor or very bad perceived health during the last year being the most likely to have mental health problems.

The results given in Table 2 present the measurements of the linear relationships between the total score obtained in the test and the risk factors (sex, age, occupational class and perceived health).

Risk factors explain 5.5% of the variability of the total score of the SDQ, but the influence of all of them is very significant, together (test $F = 40.007$) and separately (t-statistic).

On the other hand, taking into account the risk factors arises the interest in calculating the odds ratios and relative risks of being ill or healthy (Table 3).

Table 3. Ratios and Odds Ratios depending on the different risk factors.

Risk Factor	Rate [a]	Observed		IC (95%)	χ2	*p*
		RR [b]	OR [c]			
Sex						
Male	0.094	1.169	1.187	(0.945–1.447)	2.08	0.14
Female	0.080			(0.940–1.499)		
Educational Level						
Pre-School	0.094	1.158	1.174	(0.874–1.530)	1.03	0.31
Secondary	0.081			(0.862–1.595)		
Educational Level						
Pre-School	0.093	0.997	0.997	(0.679–1.303)	0.13	0.72
Secondary	0.094			(0.651–1.341)		
Occupational Class						
Executive	0.058	0.705	0.686	(0.497–1.001)	3.91	0.99
Skilled	0.083			(0.472–0.998)		
Occupational Class						
Executive	0.058	0.560	0.533	(0.403–0.778)	12.56	<0.05
Non Skilled	0.104			(0.375–0.759)		
Perceived Health						
Very well/well	0.078	0.366	0.313	(0.276–0.486)	46.11	<0.05
Regular	0.213			(0.220–0.445)		
Perceived Health						
Very well/well	0.078	0.260	0.198	(0.132–0.514)	*	
Very bad/bad	0.300			(0.075–0.519)		

[a] Rate = Proportion in the risk factor group with presence of mental health problems; [b] Ratio Risk (RR) = Rate (1)/Rate (2); Odds (1) = present (1)/absent (1), Odds (2) = present (2)/absent (2); [c] Odds Ratio (OR) = Odds (1)/Odds (2). * Frequencies less than five or empty.

4. Discussion and Conclusions

According to the results obtained in this study, it seems that, although the sex, the age associated with the corresponding educational level, the perception of health in the last year, and the occupational class are factors that affect the total score in mental health difficulties (SDQ-Parents), it is exclusively the health over the last year and the occupational class that have the capacity to influence the distinction, at a diagnostic or screening level, between sick and healthy.

Regarding sex, boys are more likely to have higher overall mental health scores than younger women. However, these differences disappear when we use the cut-off points of healthy and sick for the Spanish population. They may have worse symptomatology, but at the time of either diagnosis or more thorough screening, it seems that there are no significant differences, as this agrees with the data obtained in the ENSE-2006 [9,25]. Although it is not the goal of this paper, other studies have shown that, when analyzing pathologies not globally, but in terms of scale, there is a greater symptomatology of behavioral disorders and externalizing symptoms in boys at an early age, and a more frequent occurrence of symptoms of eating disorders, depression and internalizing symptoms in girls as they progress toward adolescence [13,26,27].

On the other hand, if the child's educational level is taken into account, minors in the Pre-School stage are at higher risk of having mental health problems than those in primary education or secondary education, with primary education having a higher risk than Secondary Education. These results are in agreement with other studies that involved measurements of total SDQ scores of children between 6 and 18 years old, and where the highest scores were in the lowest ages [16]. Even so, the scientific literature is quite divergent with respect to the effects of age on the mental health of the minors or, in this case, of age associated with academic level [26]. However, when we analyzed the ability of this factor to discriminate between healthy or sick, which had not been carried out by previous investigations in Spain with this sample, no differences based on the educational level of the child could be observed. These results are in agreement with those obtained in the Spanish National Health Survey 2006, previous to the one analyzed here [28]. At the same time, factors such as "low parental education" may be a factor that negatively affects children's mental health, especially in the early stages (4–11), without affecting later stages at adolescence [29].

Some authors [30,31] point to socioeconomic status and parental education [32] as the most common causes of mental health problems in minors. This study shows the existence of an association between parents' lower occupational class and an increased probability of suffering mental health problems in minors. The most qualified occupational class offers a factor of protection in comparison to the unqualified working class, which is in agreement, again, with the data of the ENSE-2006 [16]. Other studies confirm the influence of parents' low occupational class on the mental health of the children in the Spanish and international population [29,33], even specifying how behavioral disorders or problems of hyperactivity, emotional problems, and peer problems increase in children that belong to these families [28,34]. It seems that occupational class and, even more, the presence of unemployment, both associated with low income, may be factors that favor the appearance of mental health problems in Spanish minors [28], having the capacity to to enhance depression in adolescent girls and alcohol abuse behaviors in boys [18,35]. At the same time, there is a positive relationship between the occupational class and quality of life, with this factor having an impact on the promotion of health problems, not only mental, but also physical [34]. In this sense, the significant differences of this study show how poor health in the last year favors the possibility of suffering mental health problems. Health perceived as good or very good is a protective factor against the occurrence of mental health problems, and this remained the same in both health surveys, 2006 and 2011 [9]. These results also coincide with other recent research that advocates the association between good mental health and good physical health [4]. This could indicate the need to analyze mental health when the child complains of a poor physical health in the last year, which would imply the relevance of primary care in health centers for the detection of mental health problems. At the same time, it seems that a poor socioeconomic situation, associated with a low occupational class, may influence not only poor mental health, but also poor physical health and lifestyle [15,36]. It therefore appears that socioeconomic status, associated with the occupational class of the parents, can influence mental health and, in turn, the physical health of minors [36,37]. Although differences in mental health problems have not been perceived in minors before and after the Spanish economic crisis [38], it does seem important to highlight how occupational class remains a determinant factor for their mental health in both periods. In fact, a low socioeconomic status is related to major mental health problems in parents and, as a result, to mental health problems in minors [9,30].

It is important to emphasize that, despite the strength of this study in carrying out a national population analysis under a rigorous methodology, it would be advisable to resolve its limitations through the use of the SDQ questionnaire together with clinical interviews offering information complementary to that obtained from the use of the questionnaire.

Thanks to the results of this study, it can be concluded that the low occupational class of the parents [39], connected with the poor health of the child in the last year [25], may be risk factors for Mental Health Problems in minors.

Although there was a decrease in the psychological and emotional problems of Spanish children between 2006 and 2012 [1,2], it is noteworthy that these factors remained relevant to the Spanish population, whether before (ENSE-2006) or during the economic crisis (ENSE-2011/12). Therefore, social policies are needed for detecting those families with these variables in order to be able to work with this population and to prevent future pathologies in mental health [2].

Author Contributions: F.F. is the principal investigator, and wrote the manuscript. I.R. and E.S. synthesized the literature, and made the translation and adaptation. F.F., E.F. and B.L. analyzed the data and contributed to discussion.

Conflicts of Interest: The authors declare no conflict of interest.

References

1. Beecham, J. Annual research review: Child and adolescent mental health interventions: A review of progress in economic studies across different disorders. *J. Child Psychol. Psychiatry* **2014**, *55*, 714–732. [CrossRef] [PubMed]
2. Kieling, C.; Baker-Henningham, H.; Belfer, M.; Conti, G.; Ertem, I.; Omigbodun, O.; Rohde, L.A.; Srinath, S.; Ulkuer, N.; Rahman, A. Child and Adolescent Mental Health Worldwide: Evidence for Action. *Lancet* **2011**, *378*, 1515–1525. [CrossRef]
3. Collishaw, S. Annual Research Review: Secular Trends in Child and Adolescent Mental Health. *J. Child Psychol. Psychiatry* **2015**, *56*, 370–393. [CrossRef] [PubMed]
4. Plass-Christl, A.; Haller, A.-C.; Otto, C.; Barkmann, C.; Wiegand-Grefe, S.; Hölling, H.; Schulte-Markwort, M.; Ravens-Sieberer, U.; Klasen, F. Parents with mental health problems and their children in a German population based sample: Results of the BELLA study. *PLoS ONE* **2017**, *12*, 1–14. [CrossRef] [PubMed]
5. Belfer, M.L. Child and Adolescent Mental Disorders: The Magnitude of the Problem across the Globe. *J. Child Psychol. Psychiatry* **2008**, *49*, 226–236. [CrossRef] [PubMed]
6. Alonso-Fernández, N.; Jiménez-García, R.; Alonso-Fernández, L.; Hernández-Barrera, V.; Palacios-Ceña, D. Mental Health and Quality of Life Among Spanish-born and Immigrant Children in Years 2006 and 2012. *J. Pediatr. Nurs.* **2017**, *36*, 103–110. [CrossRef] [PubMed]
7. Goodman, R. The Strengths and Difficulties Questionnaire: A Research Note. *J. Child Psychol. Psychiatry* **1997**, *38*, 581–586. [CrossRef] [PubMed]
8. Kovess-Masfety, V.; Husky, M.M.; Keyes, K.; Hamilton, A.; Pez, O.; Bitfoi, A.; Carta, M.; Goelitz, D.; Kuijpers, R.; Otten, R.; et al. Comparing the prevalence of mental health problems in children 6–11 across Europe. *Soc. Psychiatry Psychiatr. Epidemiol.* **2016**, *51*, 1093–1103. [CrossRef] [PubMed]
9. Fajardo-Bullón, F.; León, B.; Felipe-Castaño, E.; Santos, E.J. Mental Health in the Age Group 4–15 Years Based on the Results of the National Survey of Health 2006. *Rev. Esp. Salud Publica* **2012**, *86*, 445–451. [PubMed]
10. Ortuño-Sierra, J.; Fonseca-Pedrero, E.; Aritio-Solana, R.; Velasco, A.M.; de Luis, E.C.; Schumann, G.; Lawrence, C. New evidence of factor structure and measurement invariance of the SDQ across five European nations. *Eur. Child Adolesc. Psychiatry* **2015**, *24*, 1523–1534. [CrossRef] [PubMed]
11. Ministerio de Sanidad Servicios Sociales e Igualdad, and Insituto Nacional de Estadística. Encuesta Nacional de Salud 2011–2012. Instituto Nacional de Estadística, 2013. Available online: https://www.msssi.gob.es/estadEstudios/estadisticas/encuestaNacional/encuesta2011.htm (accessed on 1 May 2017).
12. Barriuso-Lapresa, L.M.; Hernando-Arizaleta, L.; Rajmil, L. Reference values of the Strengths and Difficulties Questionnaire (SDQ) version for parents in the Spanish population, 2006. *Actas Esp. Psiquiatr.* **2014**, *42*, 43–48. [PubMed]
13. Ortuño-Sierra, J.; Fonseca-Pedrero, E.; Inchausti, F.; Sastre i Riba, S. Assesing behavioural and emotional dificulties in the child adolescent population: The strengths and difficulties questionnaire (SDQ). *Papeles Psicol.* **2016**, *37*, 14–26.
14. Perou, R.; Bitsko, R.H.; Blumberg, S.J.; Pastor, P.; Ghandour, R.M.; Gfroerer, J.C.; Hedden, S.L.; Crosby, A.E.; Visser, S.N.; Schieve, L.A.; et al. Mental Health Surveillance among Children—United States, 2005–2011. *Morb. Mortal. Wkly. Report. Surveill. Summ.* **2013**, *62*, 1–35.
15. Rajmil, L.; Fernández de Sanmamed, M.J.; Choonara, I.; Faresjö, T.; Hjern, A.; Kozyrskyj, A.L.; Lucas, P.J.; Raat, H.; Séguin, L.; Spencer, L.; et al. Impact of the 2008 Economic and Financial Crisis on Child Health: A Systematic Review. *Int. J. Environ. Res. Public Health* **2014**, *11*, 6528–6546. [CrossRef] [PubMed]
16. Fajardo-Bullón, F.; León, B.; Felipe-Castaño, E.; Polo, M.I.; Santos, E.J. Salud mental en menores españoles. Variables socioeducativas. *Salud Ment.* **2015**, *38*, 329–335. [CrossRef]
17. Alegría, M.; Bijl, R.V.; Lin, E.; Walters, E.E.; Kessler, R.C. Income differences in persons seeking outpatient treatment for mental disorders: A comparison of the United States with Ontario and The Netherlands. *Arch. Gen. Psychiatry* **2000**, *57*, 383–391. [CrossRef] [PubMed]
18. Fernández-Rivas, A.; González-Torres, M.A. The Economic Crisis in Spain and Its Impact on the Mental Health of Children and Adolescents. *Eur. Child Adolesc. Psychiatry* **2013**, *22*, 583–586. [PubMed]
19. Shibata, Y.; Okada, K.; Fukumoto, R.; Nomura, K. Psychometric Properties of the Parent and Teacher Forms of the Japanese Version of the Strengths and Difficulties Questionnaire. *Brain Dev.* **2015**, *37*, 501–507. [CrossRef] [PubMed]

20. Stone, L.L.; Otten, R.; Engels, R.C.; Vermulst, A.A.; Janssens, J.M. Psychometric Properties of the Parent and Teacher Versions of the Strengths and Difficulties Questionnaire for 4- to 12-Year-Olds: A Review. *Clin. Child Fam. Psychol. Rev.* **2010**, *13*, 254–274. [CrossRef] [PubMed]
21. Goodman, A.; Goodman, R. Population Mean Scores Predict Child Mental Disorder Rates: Validating SDQ Prevalence Estimators in Britain. *J. Child Psychol. Psychiatry* **2011**, *52*, 100–108. [CrossRef] [PubMed]
22. Gómez-Beneyto, M.; Nolasco, A.; Moncho, J.; Pereyra-Zamora, P.; Tamayo-Fonseca, N.; Munarriz, M.; Salazar, J.; Tabarés-Seisdedos, R.; Girón, M. Psychometric Behaviour of the Strengths and Difficulties Questionnaire (SDQ) in the Spanish National Health Survey 2006. *BMC Psychiatry* **2013**, *13*. [CrossRef] [PubMed]
23. Rodríguez-Hernández, P.J.; Betancort, M.; Ramírez-Santana, G.M.; García, R.; Sanz-Álvarez, E.J.; De las Cuevas-Castresana, C. Psychometric Properties of the Parent and Teacher Versions of the Strength and Difficulties Questionnaire (SDQ) in a Spanish Sample. *Int. J. Clin. Health Psychol.* **2012**, *12*, 265–279.
24. Domingo-Salvany, A.; Regidor, E.; Alonso, J.; Alvarez-Dardet, C. Una Propuesta de Medida de La Clase Social. *Atención Primaria* **2000**, *25*, 350–363. [PubMed]
25. Ortuño-Sierra, J.; Fonseca-Pedrero, E.; Paíno, M.; Aritio-Solana, R. Prevalence of emotional and behavioral symptomatology in Spanish adolescents. *Rev. Psiquiatr. Salud Ment.* **2014**, *7*, 121–130. [CrossRef] [PubMed]
26. Arman, S.; Keypour, M.; Maracy, M.R.; Attari, A. Epidemiological Study of Youth Mental Health Using Strengths and Difficulties Questionnaire (SDQ). *Iran Red Crescent Med. J.* **2012**, *14*, 371–375. [CrossRef] [PubMed]
27. Afifi, M. Gender Differences in Mental Health. *Singapore Med. J.* **2007**, *48*, 385–391. [PubMed]
28. Arroyo-Borrell, E.; Renart, G.; Saurina, C.; Saez, M. Influence Maternal Background Has on Children's Mental Health. *Int. J. Equity Health* **2017**, *16*, 63. [CrossRef] [PubMed]
29. Sonego, M.; Llácer, A.; Galán, I.; Simón, F. The Influence of Parental Education on Child Mental Health in Spain. *Qual. Life Res.* **2013**, *22*, 203–211. [CrossRef] [PubMed]
30. Banyard, V.; Hamby, S.; Grych, J. Health effects of adverse childhood events: Identifying promising protective factors at the intersection of mental and physical well-being. *Child Abus Negl.* **2017**, *65*, 88–98. [CrossRef] [PubMed]
31. Perna, L.; Bolte, G.; Mayrhofer, H-.; Spies, G.; Mielck, A. The Impact of the Social Environment on Children's Mental Health in a Prosperous City: An Analysis with Data from the City of Munich. *BMC Public Health* **2010**, *10*, 199. [CrossRef] [PubMed]
32. Richter, M.; Moor, I.; van Lenthe, F.J. Explaining socioeconomic differences in adolescent self-rated health: The contribution of material, psychosocial and behavioural factors. *J. Epidemiol. Community Health* **2012**, *66*, 691–697. [CrossRef] [PubMed]
33. Klanšček, H.; Žiberna, J.; Korošec, A.; Zurc, J.; Albreht, T. Mental Health Inequalities in Slovenian 15-Year-Old Adolescents Explained by Personal Social Position and Family Socioeconomic Status. *Int. J. Equity Health* **2014**, *13*, 26. [CrossRef] [PubMed]
34. Potijk, M.R.; de Winter, A.F.; Bos, A.F.; Kerstjens, J.M.; Reijneveld, S.A. Behavioural and Emotional Problems in Moderately Preterm Children with Low Socioeconomic Status: A Population-Based Study. *Eur. Child Adolesc. Psychiatry* **2015**, *24*, 787–795. [CrossRef] [PubMed]
35. Barriuso-Lapresa, L.; Hernando-Arizaleta, L.; Rajmil, L. Social Inequalities in Mental Health and Health-Related Quality of Life in Children in Spain. *Pediatrics* **2012**, *130*, e528–e535. [CrossRef] [PubMed]
36. Iguacel, I.; Michels, N.; Fernández-Alvira, J.M.; Bammann, K.; De Henauw, S.; Felső, R.; Gwozdz, W.; Hunsberger, M.; Reisch, L.; Russo, P.; et al. Associations between Social Vulnerabilities and Psychosocial Problems in European Children. Results from the IDEFICS Study. *Eur. Child Adolesc. Psychiatry* **2017**. [CrossRef] [PubMed]
37. Reiss, F. Socioeconomic inequalities and mental health problems in children and adolescents: A systematic review. *Soc. Sci. Med.* **2013**, *90*, 24–31. [CrossRef] [PubMed]
38. Rajmil, L.; Siddiqi, A.; Taylor-Robinson, D.; Spencer, N. Understanding the Impact of the Economic Crisis on Child Health: The Case of Spain. *Int. J. Equity Health* **2015**, *14*, 95. [CrossRef] [PubMed]
39. Basterra, V. Percentage of psychoemotional problems in Spanish children and adolescents. Differences between 2006 and 2012. *Med. Clin. Barc.* **2016**, *147*, 393–396. [CrossRef] [PubMed]

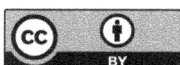

Article

Mental Health Literacy Content for Children of Parents with a Mental Illness: Thematic Analysis of a Literature Review

Joanne Riebschleger [1,*], Christine Grové [2], Daniel Cavanaugh [1] and Shane Costello [2]

1 School of Social Work, Michigan State University, 655 Auditorium Rd., East Lansing, MI 48824-1118, USA; cavana63@msu.edu
2 Faculty of Education, Monash University, 57 Scenic Blvd., Clayton, VIC 3800, Australia; christine.grove@monash.edu (C.G.); shane.costello@monash.edu (S.C.)
* Correspondence: riebsch1@msu.edu; Tel.: +01-517-353-9746

Received: 1 August 2017; Accepted: 16 October 2017; Published: 26 October 2017

Abstract: Millions of children have a parent with a mental illness (COPMI). These children are at higher risk of acquiring behavioural, developmental and emotional difficulties. Most children, including COPMI, have low levels of mental health literacy (MHL), meaning they do not have accurate, non-stigmatized information. There is limited knowledge about what kind of MHL content should be delivered to children. The aim of this exploratory study is to identify the knowledge content needed for general population children and COPMI to increase their MHL. A second aim is to explore content for emerging children's MHL scales. Researchers created and analyzed a literature review database. Thematic analysis yielded five main mental health knowledge themes for children: (1) attaining an overview of mental illness and recovery; (2) reducing mental health stigma; (3) building developmental resiliencies; (4) increasing help-seeking capacities; and (5) identifying risk factors for mental illness. COPMI appeared to need the same kind of MHL knowledge content, but with extra family-contextual content such as dealing with stigma experiences, managing stress, and communicating about parental mental illness. There is a need for MHL programs, validated scales, and research on what works for prevention and early intervention with COPMI children.

Keywords: mental illness; mental health; parents; children; prevention; mental health literacy; behavioral health

1. Introduction

There are millions of children that have a parent with a mental illness. For example, between 21% to 23% of young Australians have a parent with a mental illness [1]. England and Sim [2] explored several large health care databases to find that over 7.5 million American parents had a diagnosis of major depression. These parents had over 15 million minor children. Over 12.1% of Canadian children under 12 years of age are reported to live in households with an adult diagnosed with one or more mood, anxiety, or substance abuse disorders; one of ten children live with a parent with a mental illness [3]. Five to ten percent of British non-elderly adults are parents with mental health challenges [4]. Aldridge and Becker [5] claim that up to 30% of young carers in Great Britain have parents with mental health problems.

In this study, mental illness is identified as a disorder such as major depression, bipolar disorder, and schizophrenia [6]. Children of a parent with a mental illness (COPMI) are at higher risk of developing a mental health issue, compared to same age peers [7]. Given the prevalence and risks for these children, it is important that there are appropriate and accessible supports and interventions available to them. Most of these interventions aim to provide mental health literacy (MHL) and knowledge about their parents' illness to young people. Even though there are interventions that include educational information about parental mental health, few validated scales measure the effectiveness or efficacy of MHL in prevention interventions for children of parent with a mental illness. Indeed, there appears to be little consensus about what types of questions should be included in such outcome measures.

1.1. Risk and Resilience

Risk and resilience theories anchor the study reported herein. Early seminal studies conducted by Rutter and colleagues provided the groundwork for the later development of a risk and resiliency theory specifically to explain the needs of children exposed to parental psychiatric disabilities [8–10]. The core assumption of risk and resiliency theory can be summarized as such: exposure to high levels of biopsychosocial childhood adversity may lead to the development of future mental health difficulties [9,10]. Examples of this adversity include poor relationships in the social environment (with parents and/or peers), neighborhood violence, and exposure to parental disabilities [9]. However, there are also resiliency promoting, ameliorating factors that may reduce the likelihood that the child will experience poor developmental outcomes or future psychopathology. These include the presence of supportive relationships, coping skills, positive relationships between parents, and higher socio-economic status. Resiliency comes from learning how to handle risk with appropriate support or coping skills. Children exposed to risk in small doses may become better adjusted to dealing with future adversity [9]. However, when risk is overwhelming and omnipresent, the developing child is unable to build resistance and may face increased mental health and behavioral difficulties. These factors of risk and resiliency are composed of real, observable, events and processes that should be studied and operationalized for the creation of future interventions and prevention programs that can improve child developmental outcomes. Increasing resiliency through improved coping, elevated self-esteem, and innoculative exposure to tolerable levels of risk will help children navigate future challenges and adversity [9,11]. Risk and resilience provide further clarity by conceptualizing by considering not just specific negative or positive life occurrences, but the ongoing developmental processes that can be encouraged throughout childhood [9]. Knowledge content can be further operationalized and encouraged to promote improved developmental outcomes for children through prevention programs [12,13].

1.2. Children of a Parent with a Mental Illness

Children can be strongly impacted by parental mental illness. They are at a higher risk of developing behavioural, developmental, and emotional difficulties, compared to their same age peers [14]. Specific outcomes include increased dropout rates at school [15], a higher likelihood of being taken into foster or kinship care [16], and potentially developing a substance abuse disorder [17]. In addition, children of parents with a mental illness may enter out of home care if their parent is hospitalised and/or seriously unwell [18]. Children said they were sensitive to their parents 'good' and 'bad' days, at times reacting to parental behaviours with shame and embarrassment [19]. Similarly, Riebschleger [20] described the results from individual interviews and a focus group of children of a parent with a mental illness' experiences with their parents' good and bad days of mental health. Children defined good days as times of increased interaction, communication, and parental work and chore completion [20]. Bad days were described as times where parents were less attentive, grumpier, or more likely to yell [20].

Children of parents with a mental illness usually do not receive enough information about their parent's mental health [19,21]. They and are left 'guessing' or 'figuring out' what is happening to their parent. Children may develop misconceptions about mental illness such as blaming themselves for their parent's illness, or believing the mental illness can be caught like a cold and can be passed unto friends [18,22]. Adverse outcomes from a lack of open discussion about mental illness have also been described in the literature [23]. Keeping secrets from children is thought to lead to confusion for them [23]. Topics related to the illness may be 'off limits' for children to discuss so that there is limited or no parent-child communication about mental illness. Additionally, children may struggle to understand or worry about the parent's behaviors or they may disengage, perhaps leading their parents to believe that they are not aware of the illness [23]. Children described how a lack of mental health information caused misunderstandings and misattributions about the causes and reasons for hospital treatment and parental behavior [19,24]. Riebschleger [20] reported that children tended to describe mental health disorders by their observations of parents' behaviors. Only some children were able to provide the mental illness diagnostic label or had been specifically told about their parent's mental illness [20].

Children described increased feelings of worry when they had limited information about their parent's mental illness [25]. Without access to accurate, non-stigmatized mental health information, many children seemed to look for their own understanding of parental behaviours, often leading to confusion and distress [26]. Interviews with 20 children aged 8–22 years in Norway suggested most children were acutely aware of how their parent's behaviour, which, at times, the children associated with feeling embarrassed, ashamed, or left out [27].

Giving a child insight and knowledge into mental illness and their parent's difficulties is a key resilience factor within the literature [28]. Mental health literacy knowledge, especially when combined with social support, may serve as a protective factor for children who lack information and understanding of their parent's mental illness. For example, the mental health knowledge may help children interpret their parent's behaviour as stemming from a brain-based physical health illness that can get better [13].

1.3. Mental Health Literacy

Mental health literacy has been studied in the adult mental health literature for several decades. Mental Health Literacy (MHL) is defined as one's level of understanding about mental health attitudes and conditions, as well as one's ability to prevent, recognize, and cope with these conditions [29,30]. There are numerous mental health literacy programs, sometimes called psychoeducational programs, that aim to increase awareness of mental health challenges and facts for the general public, community crisis responders, college students, family members of adult mental health services users, and people that participate in services at mental health services agencies [30–35].

Anderson and Pierce [36] note that mental health literacy programs for adults focus on increasing mental health knowledge, confidence about helping others experiencing mental illness symptoms, as well as decreasing participants' stigmatizing attitudes toward people with mental illness. O'Connor and Casey [34] developed mental health literacy scale items for adult mental health literacy program outcomes; they included criteria related to the recognition of mental health disorders. They also included knowledge of help-seeking, mental health risk factors/causes, self-treatments (such as coping behaviors), professional help resources, and how to get help when one recognizes mental health symptoms [34].

There is some demonstrated efficacy in the use of mental health literacy (MHL) in mental health prevention and early intervention programs designed for children of parents with mental illness [28,37,38]. For example, Solantaus et al. [39] suggest that family conversations about mental health literacy can serve as preventive interventions for children of parents with depression. Kelly et al. [40] call mental health literacy interventions for adolescents "a strategy to facilitate early intervention for mental disorders".

Currently, there are a number of emerging interventions that aim to promote mental health literacy and wellbeing for children of parents with a mental illness. These include peer support groups [41], parenting or family-focused programs that focus on the parent-child connection [39], online support programs [42], school-based mental health literacy interventions [43], and bibliotherapy, i.e., including psycho-educational materials such as a DVD [44]. Canadian schools have demonstrated success in the implementation of school wide psychoeducational programs to improve the mental health literacy of their student bodies [45,46]. Programs focusing on parenting can be strong interventions to promote recovery and well-being in children and families that encounter parental mental illness [47].

These interventions are set within the much broader context of mental health promotion. Mental health promotion programs target a specific mental health challenges and populations at risk for acquiring these challenges. They use positive-psychology, strengths-based approaches to increase individual and community resilience and well-being [48]. A collaborative research group, with support from the World Health Organization, found strong evidence that mental health promotion and prevention programs are effective in enhancing public policy, creating supportive environments, strengthening community action, reorienting health services to include illness prevention, and developing personal skills such as resilience, social competence, and coping among children at risk for mental illness [49]. Interventions promoting children's protective and resiliency factors aim to influence positive developmental outcomes for at risk children [12,50]. Given these findings as well as the prevalence of and associated risks for children of parents with a mental illness, it is important that interventions are developed to prevent and reduce the transmission of mental illness in families.

A review by Reupert et al. [51] of the programs for children of a parent with a mental illness described interventions, including: family-intervention programs, peer-support programs, online interventions, and biblio-therapy. A key ingredient of these programs was psycho-education. However, well-developed and tested children's mental health literacy scales appear scarce [52]. The lack of valid and reliable child mental health literacy quantitative measures undermines the development and evaluation of evidence-based prevention programs for children of parents with a mental illness. Mental health interventions vary in their aims, evidence bases, and how they were developed. This could mean that the children of a parent with a mental illness may be less likely to receive services since funders often require programs they support to be included among databases of evidence-based practices. Resiliency is also measured using specific scales, personality inventories, and mental health literacy scales [34,53]. Thus, it is reasonable to consider that researchers compare children's levels of risk and resiliency traits with these scales before and after interventions to assess for intervention outcomes.

Clearly, scales with robust psychometric properties are a critical and often under-resourced aspect of prevention program development and evaluation in programs for children of parents with a mental illness. Strong children's mental health literacy measures are needed to help build evidence-based programs for children's mental health literacy. Therefore, this thematic analysis literature review may demonstrate a step towards addressing this gap in scale construction. This paper aims to identify mental health literacy content that may be useful to inform the development of scales to evaluate the efficacy of mental health literacy mental interventions for children of parents with a mental illness. The work is guided by a research question that asks, "What does the literature indicate are children's specific mental health knowledge needs about their parent's mental illness?"

2. Materials and Methods

The study approach combined a literature review with qualitative thematic analysis, sometimes called generic qualitative analysis [54]. Qualitative thematic analysis is a flexible research method to identify ideas and patterns presented within qualitative data [55]. It is used when other forms of qualitative methods are not a good fit for the proposed work. For example, the research may not lend itself to the "prolonged engagement" needed for phenomenological methods [54,56]. This study is particularly aligned with the work of Onwuegbuzie et al. [57], who recommended combining literature reviews with qualitative methods, including theme analyses.

2.1. Procedures

We began by defining the problem as a need to identify the themes and content that comprise children's mental health literacy. Our theoretical framework held that mental health literacy information may decrease risk and increase resilience for children of a parent with a mental illness.

We used a number of literature sources to generate search keywords. These were drawn from university e-journal library database inquiries within ProQuest, Medline and Google Scholar. Keywords were also developed from words found in written responses of COPMI experts to a survey distributed previously by the authors herein. Key words and phrases were sometimes combined to elicit mental health literacy information specific to children, and especially children of parents with a mental illness. Keywords included: "parent mental illness", "children (or child) of a parent with mental illness" and "child mental health literacy, knowledge, or information". These phrases were combined with additional keywords including parent, family, stigma, resiliency, research, program, instrument, scale and/or measure.

Inclusion criteria included English language full text peer-reviewed journal articles focused on children under age 18 with some content about the mental health knowledge needs of children. We did include general child population mental health literacy program and/or scale articles because the content would include delivery to children of parents with a mental illness within schools and community programs. However, we especially looked to include the literature-identified needs and resources for children of parents with a mental illness. We accepted some articles pertaining to children of parents with mental illness knowledge needs; prevention and early intervention program evaluations for children of parents with a mental illness; and emerging child mental health literacy scales.

We excluded duplicate articles, non-English articles, those that focused on adults (18 years and older), and adult knowledge needs, programs, and MHL scales. We excluded articles that did not target mental health specifically. For example, a health literacy article with authors' recommending teaching children about juvenile diabetes showed up in the search.

The initial pool of 238 articles was reduced to 61 after the inclusion and exclusion criteria were applied. The reasons for exclusion were that the articles focused on adult mental health consumers/patients ($n = 61$), child mental health problems ($n = 35$), services system collaboration needs ($n = 20$), only physical health ($n = 24$), and workforce preparation ($n = 11$). In addition, articles were excluded when they were repeated articles ($n = 22$), were not peer reviewed ($n = 3$), or for other reasons ($n = 3$). After initial selection of the articles, two more were excluded for having research more pertinent to adults, yielding a final number of 59 articles.

Two or more investigators read each article and independently completed a research study questionnaire form developed by the research team. The research study questionnaire was consistent with the recommendations of Beach et al. [58] for health care educational intervention literature reviews. Items on the questionnaire form included the article source (location, type and description), study methodology (study design, sampling, data collection, data analyses, limitations), and study findings. Data were collected on the sources' recommendations of the kinds of knowledge constructs needed by children of a parent with a mental illness and how that information should be provided, i.e., by whom, what content, when to talk to the children, where to talk to the children, and how to communicate the content to children.

The thematic data analysis was drawn from the review form content with article descriptions of the problem, methods, findings, and recommendations. When a study included any kind of measurement of children of parents with a mental illness mental health knowledge, the investigators captured indepth information about the scale content, such as the name, type of instrument, description, origin, use, norming sample, psychometrics and especially the specific constructs measured with the instrument. The final database file comprised 125 pages of text.

2.2. Data Analysis

Thematic analysis guided the data analysis process [55]. In regular team conference calls, each article was discussed and compared as one data source with particular exploration of the child mental health literacy content ideas emerging from the data. Decision making was by discussion and consensus. Notes were prepared from team calls and became part of the data triangulation process [56].

After many reviews and discussions, each of the researchers independently developed their "top" five to seven themes. These were inserted in a shared Dropbox folder. After reviewing the folder content, the investigators collaborated to discuss the development of each theme. There were 11 main themes initially developed by the investigators. Two were the same idea portrayed with different words and were thus condensed to one agreed-upon theme. Four of the themes were included as subthemes within the operational definition of main themes. Their constructs were integrated into the operational definition of the final main theme. One was discarded by team agreement because it was more adult-focused.

Operationalized theme definitions and early coding rules began to emerge within research team discussions [59]. For example, the team discovered the need for a shared view of recovery so as to code similarly. At times, the group explored the cultural meanings of particular words that could different implications across American, European, Canadian and Australian contexts. The group also worked through discipline specific differences in orientation and training, as the team was comprised of social workers, psychologists, and behavioral health experts. One idea they agreed to accept was a consumer and family member orientation to mental illness and holistic recovery consisting of not only medical model medication plus counseling, but also mental health consumer empowerment, nutrition, exercise, work, hobbies, relaxation exercises, and social support. This was a broader conceptualisation of recovery for some members of the team but is consistent with consumer- and family-oriented recovery models of care [60,61].

Two experienced qualitative investigators independently coded, and then compared, their responses to the completed article questionnaires. They examined the extent that the data aligned, or did not align, with one or more the five main themes. The process identified further main theme construct definition criteria and coding rules. For example, a sentence on program evaluations for children of parents with a mental illness listed mental health stigma and coping in the same excerpt but since the article was primarily devoted to mental health stigma reduction, this became the primary theme. Similarly and systematically, the coders determined the content sorting into main themes for all of the 59 articles in the full database. The data were discussed, clarified, recorded and added to the operationalized definitions of the themes and their coding rules. For example, the conceptualisation of mental illness stigma was comprised of negative assumptions about people with a mental illness based only on their mental illness diagnoses, and was expanded to include anti-mental illness "attitudes" and social distance. These enhanced definitions and coding rules created a project codebook that listed the coding rules and definitions for each theme identified [56].

The researchers used another method to increase the trustworthiness of qualitative data. They completed inter-rater reliability rates by independently rating and then comparing excerpts of text for the extent of agreement with particular themes. Development of all five themes was subject to this process. Identification of the main theme aligning with particular text excerpts yielded a 90% inter-rater reliability level. Identification of other possible themes yielded a 75% inter-rater agreement level.

3. Results

The results are reported by a general description of the mental health knowledge themes drawn from the articles in the database. It took considerable searching to yield articles pertaining to the knowledge needs of children of a parent with a mental illness. Current knowledge of children's needs for information and support seems to be much less developed than knowledge for parental mental illness. For example, a Google Scholar search for "parental mental illness" yielded over 668,000 articles compared to 112 articles generated for "children of a parent with a mental illness". While there were, at times, some overlap, the articles tended to fall into one of three article focus categories, i.e., children's needs assessments ($n = 29$), children's program evaluations ($n = 24$), and evolving children's mental health knowledge scales ($n = 6$).

3.1. Children's Mental Health Knowledge Needs

Needs assessment article authors purported that children, especially children of a parent with a mental illness, need key mental health literature information. Three articles were policy summaries focused on knowledge and support for children and families as means of preventing the onset of mental health disorders among children of a parent with a mental illness [62–64]. Five sources used COPMI group and individual interviews to gather qualitative data about children's experiences of living with a parent with a mental illness and their specific needs for information and support [13,65–68]. Several discussed how it important it is to appreciate the strengths and capacities of children of a parent with a mental illness [69,70]. Two articles examined children's needs for parental attachment [71,72]. Several used population surveys to assess children of a parent with a mental illness' risk of mental illness reported as elevated or "persistently high" [35,73].

Some of the information needs of children of parents with a mental illness included: to learn what a mental illness is [19], the different types of mental illness [68]; the causes of mental illness [74]; finding out if the parent is likely to get better or prognosis [14]; learning how to cope with the parental illness symptom fluxes [14]; and where to seek help and support [25]. Children also said they could benefit from learning what goes on in mental health services, and how to communicate with others about their parent's illness [20].

It is also important to note that exhaustive literature reviews comparing a majority of mental health literacy measures have recently been conducted [75,76]. The researchers found 89 validated measures that covered one of three mental health literacy constructs; help-seeking, stigma or mental health knowledge [77]. Most of the measures were for stigma and omitted other components of mental health literacy. Additionally, there were only four knowledge measures appropriate for children and adolescents [78]. While comprising important new knowledge development, it does not appear that any of the reviewed measures were drawn from research especially directed towards COPMI.

3.2. Evaluations of Programs for Children of Parents with a Mental Illness

Among the program evaluations, several were a literature review of summative and formative descriptions of current mental health literacy programs [50,79]. Most were descriptions of specific mental health knowledge enhancement programs for children in general; some were focused on children of parents with a mental illness. Among the 29 program evaluation sources, four employed intervention and wait-list control groups with pre, post, and follow up outcome assessment [12,41,45,80]. For example, Perry et al. [80] randomly assigned general population schoolchildren to a mental health psycho-educational intervention while others remained in their regular academic courses. For the most part, these studies revealed decreased mental health stigma as the main outcome for program children.

Most of the programs included mixed methods designs that included children of parents with a mental illness oral or written input about their learning in response to open-ended questions, plus the addition of some kind of quantitative measures, including program-developed questions that asked children to report their levels of awareness about mental illness and recovery [81,82]. Some used additional standardized scales to assess the participants functioning such as a depression scale, a hope scale, and/or a coping scale [13,39,66]. Four of the programs used a family approach where children participated in a talk about the parental mental illness [39,83,84], or in setting family goals [82]. In general, family communication about parental mental illness was improved.

Many of the programs were peer-focused; professionals provided mental health information to children of a parent with a mental illness [12,13,67,81,85–87]. One program used a DVD and a follow-up conversation to provide mental health information to children of parents with a mental illness [37]. Numerous articles described school-based interventions to teach children about mental health; many of these programs particularly focused on reducing mental illness stigma [80,88–92]. Finally, Jorm [93] used telephone interviews to find out the extent young Australians were aware of mental health organizations that provide supportive mental health information programs and direct services; unfortunately, many of the interviewees had little knowledge of the available programs.

Gladstone et al. [19] suggest that psycho-education programs should attempt to include young people's views of their parent's illness and should recognise the children's roles within the family context. Additionally, children may want help with practical issues such as providing support when their parent is hospitalised and when they need a break from caring for their parent [18,22,74].

3.3. Emerging Children's Mental Health Literacy Scales

There was significant overlap between program evaluation and emerging children's mental health literacy scales. While 15 articles described the use of quantitative measures of mental health literacy, six of these were designed to measure program-specific learning rather than mental health literacy more broadly. Of the remaining measures of mental health literacy, several were used in only one article. Two measures appeared in two articles. The first appeared in Wahl and colleagues in 2011 and 2012 [43,91]. The second appeared in Fraser and Packenham in 2008 and 2009 [12,94]. Finally, another measure appeared in three articles [37,44,95].

A variety of question types were used in the children's mental health literacy measures. The most common type of question was a multiple choice [13,37,44,80,89,94–96]. Several measures used open-ended questions, with participants receiving higher scores for more accurate responses [87,92,94,96]. Two measures used a multiple choice format, where more accurate responses were scored higher [43,91]. Two measures used vignettes to present contextual scenarios [96,97]. All measures were comparatively brief, with a median length of seven questions per measure, ranging from five to 28 items.

Generally, little detail was provided about the measures themselves. With the exception of test-retest reliability [43,91], and internal consistency [43,89], no other psychometric data were reported. One article cited test-retest reliability and internal consistency for its measure from an adult sample [80], but did not report it in the child sample. No article provided evidence of convergent and discriminant validity for the measures. There was also little detail provided regarding the content of the unpublished measures.

With the exception of two measures which focused predominantly on knowledge about depression [80,97], all instruments identified as measuring mental health and illness knowledge in the broad sense. Depression-specific measures used either vignettes or multiple choice questions, which focused on the identification of symptoms such as suicidal ideation, emotional distress, loss of interest in enjoyable activities, loss of appetite and weight loss, sleep disturbance, poor concentration, and fatigue. Examples of broad mental health literacy items included "People who have had mental illness include astronauts, presidents, and famous baseball players" and "Most people with severe forms of mental illness do not get better, even with treatment" [43]. Other areas of mental health literacy reflected in the identified measures include stereotypes and beliefs [37,44,95], as well as recovery and stigma [13,96]. An example of a recovery item was "Mental health treatment usually works as well as treatment for other health problems", and a stigma item was "It is not easy to tell if someone has a psychiatric illness by looking at them" [13]. The paucity of detail regarding the content of items used to measure mental health literacy was notable, with most articles not including the measures in full or even providing sample items.

3.4. Children's Mental Health Knowledge Content Themes

Over 30 sources recommended mental health literacy programs and initiatives for increasing children's knowledge of mental illness and recovery. The thematic analysis yielded five main themes of mental health literacy for children of a parent with a mental illness These knowledge themes focused on children, especially children of a parent with a mental illness: (1) attaining an overview of mental illness and recovery; (2) reducing mental health stigma; (3) building developmental resiliencies; (4) increasing help-seeking capacities; and (5) identifying risk factors for mental illness.

Theme One: Attaining an overview of mental illness and recovery. Many of the authors of the database articles asserted that children, especially children of a parent with a mental illness, need to acquire an overview of mental illness and recovery. However, exactly what kind of information should be delivered was less clear. Across the sources, there were references to children of a parent with a mental illness needs for knowledge of mental illnesses including depression, anxiety, bipolar disorder, borderline personality disorder, schizophrenia, substance abuse, and co-occurring mental illness and substance abuse [20,46,84,97,98].

Some authors asked children to learn the symptoms of particular mental illnesses using psychiatric diagnoses behavioral criteria. For example, Wright et al. [99] examined the extent that children could recognize signs of depression and psychosis. Similarly, Lam [100] used mental health case vignettes to survey the extent that 1678 students were able to label depression and report their willingness to seek help. For the most part, it was unclear how the overview of mental illness content was to be adapted for ages of children and their levels of development. One exception is an early article by Henderson [101] that describes discussion questions for middle school COPMI students attending a school-based counseling group.

One area that seemed clearer is that some authors suggested children should learn that mental illness was a health condition and it could often get better with treatment and recovery [68,91,102]. Some suggested that children be taught that mental illness affects at least one in five people and is therefore a very common health condition that affects many people, as well their families [13]. Other than referring to "getting help" for mental illness, it was not always clear what children were told or should be told about mental health recovery. It did appear that most frequently, the authors spoke of medical model treatment of medication and counseling, followed by support, and sometimes including stress management, health habits, and life activities [13,68,88,99].

When compared with general population children such as those in school classrooms, COPMI-focused articles were more likely to identify the need for mental health literacy to contain content on family experiences of living with a person with a mental illness. For example, they identified family "good days and bad days" linked to the symptoms levels of the person with the mental illness [20]; and "navigating an unpredictable daily life" [103]. Children needed to be able to engage in problem solving for assessing how they should respond to parents on "good days" and "bad days" [20], particularly as some COPMI claim family connections and interactions vary with the cyclical nature of mental illness symptoms of a parent [98].

A number of articles contained content supporting the use of peer sharing among children of a parent with a mental illness' awareness that many other children have similar family experiences [41,68,81,85,101]. Similarly, some database sources described children of a parent with a mental illness and family experiences in having parent-led family discussions about the specific illness of the parent and family member impacts, feelings, interactions, and communication [39,51]. These could also include parental crises, episodes, hospitalizations and child-parent separations [51]. Reupert et al. [51] listed specific key messages for parents talking to their children including: children don't cause mental illness; children don't need to "fix" the parent's illness; the parent is getting help; it's okay for the child to ask questions; it's okay for the child to say how she or he feels about the illness; and there are supportive people the child can access. Additionally, Grové and colleagues [95] explained that children are not responsible for taking care of their parents; the authors emphasized the need to convey this as part of mental health literacy for children of a parent with a mental illness.

Theme two: Reducing mental health stigma. Mental health consumer parents said that their minor children received most of their knowledge about mental illness from the media; they said this led the children to have stigmatized views of people with mental illness [102]. A plethora of studies focused on mental health literacy help to reduce children's assumptions or "attitudes" that people with mental illness are incompetent, unstable, immoral, violent and people to be avoided [92]. Instead, children can learn that most people with mental illness can work, make decisions, develop their talents, and contribute to the world [36,88]. It appears that reduction of children's mental illness stigma is a main outcome of many mental health literacy programs; many of the programs reportedly challenge mental illness misconceptions [80,91,104]. Many of the program evaluation articles were drawn from pre- and post-mental health literacy program outcomes with sampling drawn from whole classrooms of general population children [43,89–92,105].

COPMI-focused sources identified a need to address general mental illness stigma as well, but with the addition of discussing stigma experiences of children in living in a family with a person with a mental illness [85,86]. This can include external sources of stigma such as teasing from peers and others; it can also include self-stigma such as being embarrassed by parental behaviors [98,103]. Mental health literacy for COPMI children can include helping children develop strategies for dealing with external and internal stigma experiences [98].

Theme three: Building developmental resiliencies. Children of a parent with a mental illness who learn how to deal with mental health stigma may demonstrate enhanced developmental resiliency in the face of child and family stigma experiences [37,65]. Access to mental health information was sometimes linked to the idea that "knowledge is power" for children of a parent with a mental illness [86]. Children exposed to accurate, non-stigmatized mental illness and recovery information reported they were able to understand their parents' behaviors, share stories with peers, talk to their parents about mental illness, and they felt less alone [86]. For example, some children reported that being able to talk about parental mental illness with peers was "like a weight off your shoulders" [86]. Social support from nurturing adults, siblings, and peers helps strengthen developmental resiliencies of children of a parent with a mental illness [85,94].

It is also important for children to have meaningful connections and attachments with parents and other caregivers [71,72]. Supported parents may build more positive and stronger relationships with their children; the quality of children's relationships with their parents is an important resiliency factor [83,98,106]. Family communication, including communication about parental mental illness, may help children of a parent with a mental illness build additional developmental resiliency [51].

Many sources described mental health literacy programs as mechanisms for prevention of mental illness for children of a parent with a mental illness [39,64,81,83]. For example, Solantaus and colleagues [39] found that children of a parent with a mental illness who participated in a family discussion about a parental mood disorder showed decreased reported emotional symptoms, anxiety, and hyperactivity, as well as increased pro-social behavior. These appear to indicate children's enhanced resiliencies.

Some of the articles discussed the need for children of parents with a mental illness to learn and practice stress management skills toward building resilient behaviors [13]. Riebschleger and colleagues [13] reported that children need to learn how to reach out to supportive people and resources; the children may need personalized, active stress management plans [68,103]. Active stress management skills are likely to decrease risks of mental illness. In addition, it is important to recognize the strengths of children of a parent with a mental illness; for example, some children of a parent with a mental illness report that they have strong skills in crisis management, problem solving, and caregiving [69,70]. It is also important that children of a parent with a mental illness learn how and when to help, or not help, others, including parents and other family members [102].

Theme four: Increasing help-seeking capacities. Many sources identified the need for children, especially children of a parent with a mental illness, to seek help for personal distress, and sometimes, parental and family crises [78,93,97,104]. In fact, some sources described mental health literacy programs as mechanisms of early intervention should mental illness symptoms appear among the children; the logic is that children are more likely to recognize mental illness symptoms and to know how to seek help [40,63]. Children who view mental illness as health condition that is no one's fault may be more likely to seek help [13]. If children, including children of a parent with a mental illness, have some basic information about recovery and think recovery can be effective, they may be more likely to seek help as well [78,96]. Further, stigma may be much less of a barrier to help-seeking for child participants of mental health literacy programs [46,91].

Some sources noted that help-seeking of children of a parent with a mental illness help-seeking should including an awareness of professional and community mental health treatment resources [93], as well as children of a parent with a mental illness reaching out to trusted adults, peers, siblings, and others [78]. A few sources mentioned COPMI help-seeking can be part of mental health knowledge areas of preparing for crisis management and safety planning [13,106].

In addition to increased child reported help-seeking capacities, numerous mental health literacy program evaluation sources indicated that child mental health literacy program participants reported they were more likely to engage in providing help to people with a mental illness. For example, Olsson and Kennedy [107] found adolescents exposed to vignette-based hypothetical situations about a peer with mental illness symptoms were able to say how they would respond, or help, the peer described in the case example. The ability to seek and provide help can be associated with higher levels of developmental functioning and resiliency. Yap and Jorm [108] surveyed 1520 Australian youth and found that subjects reporting less mental illness stigma attitudes also said they would be more likely to help a friend or family member with a mental health problem.

Theme five: Identifying risk factors for mental illness. Numerous sources identified the need for children to be able to identify possible mental health conditions, such as depression, by the duration and intensity of particular diagnostic behaviors within case examples [99,100,107]. The ability to identify early warning signs of mental illness were said to be desirable for promoting child/COPMI help-seeking behaviors [109]. Very few of the articles seemed to identify particular early warning signs [109], such as isolating oneself or persistent sadness. Some sources appeared to reference a combination of biological and environmental stressors as precipitators of the onset of mental illness symptoms [62,108]. A few sources suggested that children of a parent with a mental illness need information about heritability of mental illness [13,87]. Some sources said that children can explore factors that might help mitigate risk factors for mental illness, such as using active stress management, connecting with others, communicating with family members about mental illness, finding community resources, and engaging in good health habits [81,103]. Jorm [109] provided a list of strategies suggested for those with subclinical depression such as maintaining a good sleep schedule, engaging in exercise, learning relaxation, and doing something one enjoys. Despite elevated statistical risk factors, a few of the sources suggested there is a need for children of a parent with a mental illness to experience feelings of hope about their families and their futures [13,68].

4. Discussion

The research question asked, "What does the literature indicate are children's specific mental health knowledge needs about their parent's mental illness?" The main themes of the data were: (1) attaining an overview of mental illness and recovery; (2) reducing mental health stigma; (3) building developmental resiliencies; (4) increasing help-seeking capacities; and (5) identifying risk factors for mental illness. The findings revealed some general knowledge constructs for children as a whole, often set within classroom mental health literacy programs. Other sources focused on the additional knowledge needs of children of a parent with a mental illness.

Theme one data seemed to show that an overview of children's mental illness and recovery content included identifying specific illness behaviors and symptoms, mental illness as a health challenge, and recovery actions such as taking medications, participating in counseling, managing stress, finding support, and maintaining good health habits. A main message for children seemed to be that people could get better within mental health recovery. Information especially pertinent to children of a parent with a mental illness was the need to deal with specific family member behaviors changes from day to day, as mental illness symptom levels vacillated. Mental health literacy content on problem solving and day to day coping was recommended. The need for peer sharing and parent-led family discussions about mental illness was also advised.

Theme two data indicated that children need to know about mental health stigma. This was often presented within illustrative case vignettes. Some sources found that lower levels of mental illness stigma seemed to promote increased willingness to seek help for mental illness concerns. Children who learned about stigma and may have replaced these ideas with factual information about mental illness also seemed to report they were more willing to help peers and family members that had mental health challenges. Children of a parent with a mental illness reportedly needed to process external family stigma episodes when others teased them or their family members with a mental illness. They also had to deal with internal stigma, including how they felt about themselves and their family member's mental illness. Children of a parent with a mental illness may be able to benefit from developing strategies for responding to internal and external stigma.

Theme three reported that mental health literature revealed that is it useful for children to know how to seek help for themselves and others in the event of a mental health concern. However, theme four findings largely target children of a parent with a mental illness who may use mental illness and recovery information as a beginning step toward reducing the impact of developmental risks. For example, children could glean more knowledge of their parent's illness. They may be more likely to begin to talk to their peers and their parents about their mental illness. There was a strong recommendation within a number of database sources for children of a parent with a mental illness to engage in outreach to supportive individuals and, especially, to create and implement active stress management planning. Information for children of a parent with a mental illness should also include identification of strengths.

Theme four data seemed to indicate that children need to be able to increase their mental health help-seeking capacities. Children of a parent with a mental illness may particularly benefit from learning that mental illness is not anyone's fault and it is certainly not the children's fault. They may find there are times when they may need to seek help for their own personal distress and perhaps even family or parent crises. It is also important that children of a parent with a mental illness learn how and when to help or not help others, including parents and other family members. Some sources identified a need for the children to develop crises and safety planning.

Theme five data appear to relay that children need some information about risk factors for mental illness. Some sources said children would need to be able to identify early warning signs of mental illness. However, few sources said what these early warning signs were except to say they would be tied to particular diagnoses, such as depression. A few sources said that mental health literacy information would likely identify possible biopsychosocial influences for developing mental illness. COPMI-focused sources particularly emphasized the need for coaching these children in active stress management, connecting with others, communicating with family members, finding community resources, and engaging in good health habits.

The findings for children as a general target group, such as those used in school-based mental health literacy interventions seem to align well with the work of O'Conner and Casey [34], Wahl et al. [44,91], and McLuckie et al. [89], all of whom delivered mental health literacy programs in school classrooms. These sources seemed to consider the original work of Jorm and colleagues' original work in mental health literacy for adults [29,30,109] and with young people [93]. Specifically, they included content on a person's abilities to: recognize specific disorders, know how to seek mental health information, identify mental illness risk factors and causes, engage in self-care, know professional help resources that are available, and seek help after recognizing emerging mental illness warning signs or symptoms. In this study, the findings also indicated the need for these constructs under themes of obtaining an overview of mental illness and recovery; decreasing mental health stigma; increasing help-seeking capacities; and identifying risk factors for mental illness.

It is noted that the thematic finding of building developmental resiliencies is consistent with some of the more COPMI-focused articles such as those by Foster et al. [66,85], Gladstone et al. [67,70], Grové et al. [37,44,95], Mordoch and Hall [25], Riebschleger [20], and Riebschleger et al. [13] These needs and program assessment sources particularly focused on the interactions between children of a parent with a mental illness and their parents, peers and others. It appears that this thematic finding may support risk and resilience as a theoretical foundation for mental health literacy programs for children with a parent with a mental illness. They seem to align with Rutter's recommendations for resiliency-promoting, ameliorating factors such as children having supportive relationships, coping skills and learning how to deal with family-related emotional risk factors, such as stigma experiences [9].

4.1. Strengths and Limitations

This study has a number of limitations and strengths. A lack of detail in many of the articles sometimes made it difficult to identify the child mental health literacy content. For example, many of the articles evaluating children's mental health literacy referred to measures or scales but they did not provide scale questions. Program evaluation sources sometimes did not prove details of the program content covered. However, among those that did provide scale questions or program description, it was possible to glean some useful data about child mental health literacy content. The use of a form for the literature reviews further reduced mental health literacy content detail available. In some cases, it was necessary to go back to the original articles for more clarification. Finally, engaging in thematic analysis using literature formatted in third person and whole study perspectives was challenging. However, as indicated by Onwuegbuzie et al. [57], it was possible to engage in a thematic analysis of a literature database.

Other limitations of the study include the early level of development of the child knowledge base of mental health literacy and measurements of child mental health literacy levels. However, given the limited number of sources for children's mental health literacy and even less for mental health literacy for children of a parent with a mental illness, the researchers were still able to draw a good deal of children's mental health literacy content from COPMI needs assessment, program evaluations, and emerging scales.

The data sources herein were drawn from only three databases. It is possible that other children's mental health literacy sources were available among other databases not selected, but well-known and broad spectrum databases were used. Since only articles in English were included in the database, this remains a limitation of the study.

Qualitative studies require interpretation by research analysts, so bias can be a concern. Creswell [56] says that the trustworthiness of the data can be strengthened when the researchers use two or data collection and analysis strategies. In this study, the researchers used data triangulation, developed a code book that may be used for replicating the study, and demonstrated good inter-rater reliability for data coding.

4.2. Recommendations

With the early state of knowledge development in mind, it may still be possible to offer some modest recommendations for practice, policy and research. There appears to be a need for mental health literacy programs for children from the general population. Many of these are school-based and have demonstrated that they appear to increase knowledge of mental illness and to reduce mental health stigma among children. Children of parents with a mental illness need the same basic information with a good deal more additional information tied to family experiences with mental illness, including talking to family members about mental illness. They need accurate, non-stigmatized and family-contextual mental health literacy information. There is a need for children of a parent with a mental illness to learn how to build skills as well as knowledge for help-seeking, helping peers/family members, responding to stigma experiences, talking to peers, actively managing stress and feeling hopeful.

Since mental health literacy programs are needed for children, policy makers need to prioritize and fund the delivery of mental health knowledge to children and to children that have a parent with a mental illness. This enhances the development of manualized, evidence-based mental health literacy programs for all children and children of a parent with a mental illness. Workforce preparation is needed as well as collaboration between federal, state and community agencies that deliver health, mental health, child welfare and educational services [110]. The development of the programs should include the active participation of children of a parent with a mental illness and their parents. Support for parental roles should be further explored and supported. Recovery frames may need to be more holistic and less medical model in orientation. For example, the self-care suggestions of O'Connor and Casey [34], as well as Jorm [93], should be included, in addition to those recommended by children, parents, and other family members. It may be useful to consider the inclusion of strength-based and empowerment theories within program content and delivery processes.

Future research should be well funded to execute larger sampling and more rigorous designs. In fact, there is need to study what kind of mental health information should be available to children, at what age, and how it should be delivered. Evidence-based child mental health literacy programs will require the development of validated scales with strong psychometric properties. It may be necessary to develop children's mental health knowledge scales for particular age children. COPMI children may need additional questions specifically targeted toward their family experiences, such as dealing with stigma experiences, managing stress, and communicating about parental mental illness. The scales need to align with children's developmental levels and backgrounds. Thus, there is likely to be a need for variations of the scales by age groups, family circumstances, languages and cultural group affiliations.

5. Conclusions

It is clear that there is much work to do in order to ensure that all children, especially COPMI, have access to accurate mental health information and support. Mental health literacy programs could help increase accessibility of the information but they require mental health literacy scales and strong evaluation to show "what works" for building children with high levels of mental health literacy. Practice, policy, and research could help millions of children of a parent with a mental illness find increased family understanding, coping, and hope for their developmental futures.

Acknowledgments: We acknowledge the Educational Psychology & Inclusive Education Academic Community Research and Scholarship Stimulus Scheme 2017 at the Faculty of Education, Monash University for supporting open access of this publication.

Author Contributions: Joanne Riebschleger worked on all of the writing sections, especially the methods section. She also served as the coordinator of the manuscript development and submission. Christine Grové particularly worked on the discussion section of the manuscript and made editing suggestions throughout. Shane Costello wrote the scale topic part of the discussion section and headed up the revision of the references section to journal guidelines format. Shane Costello also provided new citations; he proofread and edited the work. Daniel Cavanaugh wrote much of the background section, provided references for the initial reference section, and proofread the document. He led much of the literature review data collection.

Conflicts of Interest: The authors declare no conflicts of interest.

References

1. Maybery, D.; Reupert, A.; Goodyear, M.; Patrick, K.; Crase, L. Prevalence of children whose parents have a mental illness. *Psychiatr. Bull.* **2009**, *33*, 22–26. [CrossRef]
2. England, M.J.; Sim, L.J. *Depression in Parents, Parenting, and Children: Opportunities to Improve Identification, Treatment, and Prevention*; National Academies Press: Washington, DC, USA, 2009.
3. Bassani, D.G.; Padoin, C.V.; Philippe, D.; Veldhuizen, S. Estimating the number of children exposed to parental psychiatric illness through a national health survey. *Child Adolesc. Psychiatry Ment. Health* **2009**, *3*, 1–7. [CrossRef] [PubMed]
4. Parker, G.; Beresford, B.; Clarke, S.; Gridley, K.; Pitman, R.; Spiers, G.; Light, K. Research Reviews on Prevalence, Detection, and Interventions in Parental Mental Health and Child Welfare: Summary Report. Available online: http://php.york.ac.uk/inst/spru/research/summs/pm (accessed on 1 April 2017).
5. Aldridge, J.; Becker, S. *Children Caring for Parents with Mental Illness: Perspectives of Young Carers, Parents, and Professionals*; Policy Press: Bristol, UK, 2003.

6. American Psychiatric Association. *Diagnostic and Statistical Manual of Mental Disorders (DSM-5®)*; American Psychiatric Association: Washington, DC, USA, 2013.

7. Edwards, E.P.; Eiden, R.D.; Leonard, K.E. Behaviour problems in 18- to 36-month-old children of alcoholic fathers: Secure mother-infant attachment as a protective factor. *Dev. Psychopathol.* **2006**, *18*, 395–407. [CrossRef] [PubMed]

8. Rutter, M. Psychosocial resilience and protective mechanisms. *Am. J. Orthopsychiatry* **1987**, *57*, 316–331. [CrossRef] [PubMed]

9. Rutter, M. Resilience: Some conceptual considerations. *J. Adolesc. Health* **1993**, *14*, 626–631. [CrossRef]

10. Rutter, M.; Quinton, D. Parental psychiatric disorder: Effects on children. *Psychol. Med.* **1984**, *14*, 853–880. [CrossRef] [PubMed]

11. Zimmerman, M.A. Resiliency theory: A strengths-based approach to research and practice for adolescent health. *Health Educ. Behav.* **2013**, *40*, 381–383. [CrossRef] [PubMed]

12. Fraser, E.; Pakenham, K.I. Evaluation of a resilience-based intervention for children of parents with mental illness. *Aust. N. Z. J. Psychiatry* **2008**, *42*, 1041–1050. [CrossRef] [PubMed]

13. Riebschleger, J.; Tableman, B.; Rudder, D.; Onaga, E.; Whalen, P. Early outcomes of a pilot psychoeducation group intervention for children of a parent with a psychiatric illness. *Psychiatr. Rehabil. J.* **2009**, *33*, 133–141. [CrossRef] [PubMed]

14. Reupert, A.E.; Maybery, D.J.; Kowalenko, N.M. Children whose parents have a mental illness: Prevalence, need and treatment. *Med. J. Aust.* **2012**, *196*, 7–9. [CrossRef]

15. Farahati, F.; Marcotte, D.E.; Wilcox-Gok, V. The effects of parents' psychiatric disorders on children's high school dropout. *Econ. Educ. Rev.* **2003**, *22*, 167–178. [CrossRef]

16. Leschied, A.W.; Chiodo, D.; Whitehead, P.C.; Hurley, D. The relationship between maternal depression and child outcomes in a child welfare sample: Implications for treatment and policy. *Child Family Soc. Work* **2005**, *10*, 281–291. [CrossRef]

17. Mowbray, C.T.; Oyserman, D. Substance abuse in children with mental illness: Risks, resiliency, and best prevention practices. *J. Prim. Prev.* **2003**, *23*, 451–483. [CrossRef]

18. Maybery, J.D.; Ling, L.; Szakacs, E.; Reupert, A.E. Children of a parent with a mental illness: Perspectives on need. *Aust. e-J. Adv. Ment. Health* **2005**, *4*, 78–88. [CrossRef]

19. Gladstone, B.M.; Boydell, K.M.; Seeman, M.V.; McKeever, P.D. Children's experiences of parental mental illness: A literature review. *Early Interv. Psychiatry* **2011**, *5*, 271–289. [CrossRef] [PubMed]

20. Riebschleger, J. Good days and bad days: The experiences of children of a parent with a psychiatric disability. *Psychiatr. Rehabil. J.* **2004**, *28*, 25–31. [CrossRef] [PubMed]

21. Monds-Watson, A.; Manktelow, R.; McColgan, M. Social work with children when parents have mental health difficulties: Acknowledging vulnerability and maintaining the "rights of the child". *Child Care Pract.* **2010**, *16*, 35–55. [CrossRef]

22. Fudge, E.; Mason, P. Consulting with young people about service guidelines relating to parental mental illness. *Aust. e-J. Adv. Ment. Health* **2004**, *3*, 50–58. [CrossRef]

23. Imber-Black, E. Eschewing certainties: The creation of family therapists in the 21st Century. *Family Process* **2014**, *53*, 371–379. [CrossRef] [PubMed]

24. Stallard, P.; Norman, P.; Huline-Dickens, K.; Salter, E.; Cribb, J. The effects of parental mental illness upon children: A descriptive study of the views of parents and children. *Clin. Child Psychol. Psychiatry* **2004**, *9*, 39–52. [CrossRef]

25. Mordoch, E.; Hall, W.A. Children's perceptions of living with a parent with a mental illness: Finding the rhythm and maintaining the frame. *Qual. Health Res.* **2008**, *18*, 1127–1144. [CrossRef] [PubMed]

26. Garley, D.; Gallop, R.; Johnston, N.; Pipitone, J. Children of the mentally ill: A qualitative focus group approach. *J. Psychiatr. Ment. Health Nurs.* **1997**, *4*, 97–103. [CrossRef] [PubMed]

27. Fjone, H.H.; Ytterhus, B.; Almvik, A. How children with parents suffering from mental health distress search for "normality" and avoid stigma. To be or not to be is not the question. *Childhood* **2009**, *16*, 461–477. [CrossRef]

28. Reupert, A.E.; Maybery, D.J. "Knowledge is Power": Educating children about their parent's mental illness. *Soc. Work Healthc.* **2010**, *49*, 630–646. [CrossRef] [PubMed]

29. Jorm, A.F.; Korten, A.E.; Jacomb, P.A.; Christensen, H.; Rodgers, B.; Pollitt, P. "Mental health literacy:" A survey of the public's ability to recognise mental disorders and their beliefs about the effectiveness of treatment. *Med. J. Aust.* **1997**, *166*, 182–186. [PubMed]

30. Jorm, A.F.; Christensen, H.; Griffiths, K.M. The public's ability to recognize mental disorders and their beliefs about treatment: Changes in Australia over 8 years. *Aust. N. Z. J. Psychiatry* **2006**, *40*, 36–41. [CrossRef] [PubMed]

31. Eker, F.; Harkin, S. Effectiveness of six-week psychoeducation program on adherence of patients with bipolar affective disorder. *J. Affect. Disord.* **2012**, *138*, 409–416. [CrossRef] [PubMed]

32. Hadlaczky, G.; Hökby, A.; Mkrtchian, A.; Carli, V.; Wasserman, D. Mental health first aid is an effective public health intervention for improving knowledge, attitudes, and behaviour: A meta-analysis. *Int. Rev. Psychiatry* **2014**, *26*, 467–475. [CrossRef] [PubMed]

33. Falloon, I.R.H. Family interventions for mental disorders: Efficacy and effectiveness. *World Psychiatry* **2003**, *2*, 20–28. [PubMed]

34. O'Connor, M.; Casey, L. The Mental Health Literacy Scale (MHLS): A new scale-based measure of mental health literacy. *Psychiatry Res.* **2015**, *229*, 511–516. [CrossRef] [PubMed]

35. Siegenthaler, E.; Munder, T.; Egger, M. Effect of preventive interventions in mentally ill parents on the mental health of the offspring: Systematic review and meta-analysis. *J. Am. Acad. Child Adolesc. Psychiatry* **2012**, *5*, 8–17. [CrossRef] [PubMed]

36. Anderson, R.J.; Pierce, D. Assumptions associated with mental health literacy training—Insights from initiatives in rural Australia. *Adv. Ment. Health* **2012**, *10*, 258–267. [CrossRef]

37. Grové, C.; Reupert, A.E.; Maybery, D.J. Gaining knowledge about parental mental illness: How does it empower children? *Child Family Soc. Work* **2015**, *20*, 377–386. [CrossRef]

38. Trondsen, M.V. Living with a mentally ill parent exploring adolescents' experiences and perspectives. *Qual. Health Res.* **2012**, *22*, 174–188. [CrossRef] [PubMed]

39. Solantaus, T.; Paavonen, E.J.; Toikka, S.; Punamäki, R.L. Preventive interventions in families with parental depression: Children's psychosocial symptoms and prosocial behaviour. *Eur. Child Adolesc. Psychiatry* **2010**, *19*, 883–892. [CrossRef] [PubMed]

40. Kelly, C.M.; Jorm, A.F.; Wright, A. Improving mental health literacy as a strategy to facilitate early intervention for mental disorders. *Med. J. Aust.* **2007**, *187*, 26–30.

41. Van Santvoort, F.; Hosman, C.M.; van Doesum, K.T.; Janssens, J.M. Effectiveness of preventive support groups for children of mentally ill or addicted parents: A randomized controlled trial. *Eur. Child Adolesc. Psychiatry* **2014**, *23*, 473–484. [CrossRef] [PubMed]

42. Drost, L.M.; Sytema, S.; Schippers, G.M. Internet support for adolescents with a mentally ill family member. *Psychiatr. Serv.* **2011**, *62*, 322. [CrossRef] [PubMed]

43. Wahl, O.; Susin, J.; Lax, A.; Kaplan, L.; Zatina, D. Knowledge and attitudes about mental illness: A survey of middle school students. *Psychiatr. Serv.* **2012**, *63*, 649–654. [CrossRef] [PubMed]

44. Grové, C.; Reupert, A.E.; Maybery, D.J. Peer connections as an intervention for young people of parents with a mental illness: Moving toward understanding the processes of change. *Child. Youth Serv. Rev.* **2015**, *48*, 177–185. [CrossRef]

45. Kutcher, S.; Bagnell, A.; Wei, Y. Mental health literacy in secondary schools: A Canadian approach. *Child Adolesc. Psychiatr. Clin. N. Am.* **2015**, *24*, 233–244. [CrossRef] [PubMed]

46. Kutcher, S.; Wei, Y.; Morgan, C. Successful application of a Canadian mental health curriculum resource by usual classroom teachers in significantly and sustainably improving student mental health literacy. *Can. J. Psychiatry* **2015**, *60*, 580–586. [CrossRef] [PubMed]

47. Reupert, A.; Price-Robertson, R.; Maybery, D. Parenting as a focus of recovery: A systematic review of current practice. *Psychiatr. Rehabil. J.* **2017**. [CrossRef] [PubMed]

48. Kobau, R.; Seligman, M.E.; Peterson, C.; Diener, E.; Zack, M.M.; Chapman, D.; Thompson, W. Mental health promotion in public health: Perspectives and strategies from positive psychology. *Am. J. Public Health* **2011**, *101*, 1–9. [CrossRef] [PubMed]

49. Jané-Llopis, E.; Barry, M.; Hosman, C.; Patel, V. Mental health promotion works: A review. *Promot. Educ.* **2005**, *12*, 1–18. [CrossRef]

50. Riebschleger, J. A world tour of intervention programs for children of a parent with a psychiatric illness. In *Vulnerable Children: Global Challenges in Education, Health, Well-Being, and Child Rights*; Johnson, D.J., Agbényiga, D.L., Hitchcock, R.K., Eds.; Springer: New York, NY, USA, 2013; pp. 141–166.

51. Reupert, A.; Cuff, R.; Maybery, D. Helping children understand their parent's mental illness. In *Parental Psychiatric Disorder: Distressed Parents and their Families*, 3rd ed.; Reupert, A., Maybery, D., Nicholson, J., Göpfert, M., Seeman, M.V., Eds.; Cambridge University Press: Cambridge, UK, 2015.

52. Reupert, A.E.; Cuff, R.; Drost, L.; Foster, K.; van Doesum, K.T.; van Santvoort, F. Intervention programs for children whose parents have a mental illness: A review. *Med. J. Aust.* **2012**, *196*, 18. [CrossRef]

53. Campbell-Sills, L.; Cohan, S.L.; Stein, M.B. Relationship of resilience to personality, coping, and psychiatric symptoms in young adults. *Behav. Res. Ther.* **2006**, *44*, 585–599. [CrossRef] [PubMed]

54. Percy, W.H.; Kostere, K.; Kostere, S. Generic qualitative research. *Qual. Rep.* **2015**, *20*, 76–85.

55. Braun, V.; Clarke, V. Using thematic analysis in psychology. *Qual. Res. Psychol.* **2006**, *3*, 77–101. [CrossRef]

56. Creswell, J.W. *Qualitative Inquiry and Research Design: Choosing among Five Approaches*, 2nd ed.; Sage: Thousand Oaks, CA, USA, 2013.

57. Onwuegbuzie, A.J.; Leech, N.L.; Collins, M.T. Qualitative analysis techniques for the review of the literature. *Qual. Rep.* **2012**, *17*, 1–28.

58. Beach, M.C.; Price, E.G.; Gary, T.L.; Robinson, K.A.; Gozu, A.; Palacio, A.; Smarth, C.; Cooper, L. Cultural competency: A systematic review of health care provider educational interventions. *Med. Care* **2005**, *43*, 356–373. [CrossRef] [PubMed]

59. Saldañas, J. *The Coding Manual for Qualitative Researchers*, 3rd ed.; Sage: Thousand Oaks, CA, USA, 2015.

60. Falkov, A. *The Family Model Handbook*; Pavillion: Teddington, UK, 2012.

61. Slade, M. *Personal Recovery and Mental Illness: A Guide for Mental Health Professionals*; Cambridge University Press: Cambridge, UK, 2009.

62. Kutcher, S.; Wei, Y.; Costa, S.; Gusmão, R.; Sokauskas, N.; Sourander, A. Enhancing mental health literacy in young people. *Eur. Child Adolesc. Psychiatry* **2016**, *25*, 567–569. [CrossRef] [PubMed]

63. McGorry, P.D.; Purcell, R.; Hickie, I.B.; Jorm, A.F. Investing in youth mental health is a best buy. *Med. J. Aust.* **2007**, *187*, S5–S7.

64. Waddell, C.; McEwan, K.; Peters, R.D.; Hua, J.M.; Garland, O. Preventing mental disorders in children: A public health priority. *Can. J. Public Health* **2007**, *3*, 174–178.

65. Bilsborrow, S. What we want from mental health professionals: "Telling it like it is". In *Parental Psychiatric Disorder: Distressed Parents and Their Families*; Reupert, A., Maybery, D., Nicholson, J., Göpfert, M., Seeman, M.V., Eds.; Cambridge University Press: Cambridge, UK, 2015; pp. 16–19.

66. Foster, K.; McPhee, I.; Fethney, J.; McCloughen, A. Outcomes of the ON FIRE peer support programme for children and adolescents in families with mental health problems. *Child Family Soc. Work* **2016**, *21*, 295–306. [CrossRef]

67. Gladstone, B.M.; McKeever, P.; Seeman, M.; Boydell, K.M. Analysis of a support group for children of parents with mental illnesses: Managing stressful situations. *Qual. Health Res.* **2014**, *24*, 1171–1182. [CrossRef] [PubMed]

68. Mordoch, E. How children understand parental mental illness: "You don't get life insurance. What's life insurance?". *J. Can. Acad. Child Adolesc. Psychiatry* **2010**, *19*, 19–25. [PubMed]

69. Drost, L.M.; van der Krieke, L.; Sytema, S.; Schippers, G.M. Self-expressed strengths and resources of children of parents with a mental illness: A systemic review. *Int. J. Ment. Health Nurs.* **2015**, *25*, 102–115. [CrossRef] [PubMed]

70. Gladstone, B.M.; Boydell, K.M.; McKeever, P. Recasting research into children's experiences of parental mental illness: Beyond risk and resilience. *Soc. Sci. Med.* **2006**, *62*, 2540–2550. [CrossRef] [PubMed]

71. Allen-Meares, P.; Blazevski, J.; Bybee, D.; Oyserman, D. Independent effects of paternal involvement and maternal mental illness on child outcomes. *Soc. Serv. Rev.* **2010**, *84*, 103–127. [CrossRef]

72. Walsh, J.; Schofield, G.; Harris, G.; Vostanis, P.; Oyebode, F.; Coulhard, H. Attachment and coping strategies in middle childhood children whose mothers have a mental health problem: Implications for social work practice. *Br. J. Soc. Work* **2009**, *39*, 81–98. [CrossRef]

73. British Medical Journal. The children of depressed parents have a persistently high risk of mental illness. *Br. Med. J.* **2006**, *333*. [CrossRef]

74. Handley, C.; Farrell, G.A.; Josephs, A.; Hanke, A.; Hazelton, M. The Tasmanian children's project: The needs of children with a parent/carer with a mental illness. *Int. J. Ment. Health Nurs.* **2001**, *10*, 221–228. [CrossRef]

75. Wei, Y.; McGrath, P.J.; Hayden, J.; Kutcher, S. Measurement properties of mental health literacy tools measuring help-seeking: A systematic review. *J. Ment. Health* **2017**, 1–13. [CrossRef] [PubMed]

76. Wei, Y.; McGrath, P.J.; Hayden, J.; Kutcher, S. Measurement properties of tools measuring mental health knowledge: A systematic review. *BMC Psychiatry* **2016**, *16*, 297–313. [CrossRef] [PubMed]

77. Wei, Y.; McGrath, P.J.; Hayden, J.; Kutcher, S. Mental health literacy measures evaluating knowledge, attitudes, and help-seeking: A scoping review. *BMC Psychiatry* **2015**, *15*, 291–311. [CrossRef] [PubMed]

78. Wei, Y.; Hayden, J.A.; Kutcher, S.; Zygmunt, A.; McGrath, P. The effectiveness of school mental health literacy programs to address knowledge, attitudes, and help-seeking among youth. *Early Interv. Psychiatry* **2013**, *7*, 109–121. [CrossRef] [PubMed]

79. Reupert, A.E.; Maybery, D.J. A "snapshot" of Australian programs to support children and adolescents whose parents have a mental illness. *Psychiatr. Rehabil. J.* **2009**, *33*, 125–132. [CrossRef] [PubMed]

80. Perry, Y.; Petrie, K.; Buckley, H.; Cavanaugh, L.; Clarke, D.; Winslade, M.; Christensen, H. Effects of a classroom-based education resource on adolescent mental health literacy: A cluster randomized controlled trial. *J. Adolesc.* **2014**, *37*, 1143–1151. [CrossRef] [PubMed]

81. Goodyear, M.; Cuff, R.; Maybery, D.; Reupert, A. Champs: A peer support program for children of parents with a mental illness. *Aust. e-J. Adv. Ment. Health* **2009**, *8*, 296–304. [CrossRef]

82. Maybery, D.; Reupert, A.; Goodyear, M. Goal setting in recovery: Families where a parent has a mental illness or a dual diagnosis. *Child Family Soc. Work* **2013**, *20*, 354–363. [CrossRef]

83. Beardslee, W.R.; Solantaus, T.; Morgan, B.S.; Gladstone, T.R.; Kowalenko, N. Preventive interventions for children of parents with depression: International perspectives. *Med. J. Aust.* **2012**, *1*, 23–25. [CrossRef]

84. Mason, W.A.; Haggerty, K.P.; Fleming, A.P.; Casey-Goldstein, M. Family intervention to prevent depression and substance use among adolescents of depressed parents. *J. Child Family Stud.* **2012**, *21*, 891–905. [CrossRef] [PubMed]

85. Foster, K.; Lewis, P.; McCloughen, A. Evaluation of a resilience-based intervention and adolescents whose parents and siblings have mental illness. *J. Child Adolesc. Psychiatr. Nurs.* **2014**, *27*, 61–67. [CrossRef] [PubMed]

86. Grové, C.; Melrose, H.; Reupert, A.E.; Maybery, D.J.; Morgan, B. When your parent has a mental illness: Children's experiences of a psycho-educational interventions. *Adv. Ment. Health* **2015**, *13*, 127–138. [CrossRef]

87. Pitman, E.; Matthey, S. The SMILES program: A group program for children with mentally ill parents or si0blings. *Am. J. Orthopsychiatry* **2004**, *74*, 383–388. [CrossRef] [PubMed]

88. Joyce, A.; Allchin, B.; Malmborg, J.; Canday, L.; Cowling, V. Primary schools: Opportune settings for changing attitudes and promoting mental health. *Health Promot. J. Aust.* **2003**, *14*, 216–218.

89. McLuckie, A.; Kutcher, S.; Wei, Y.; Weaver, C. Sustained improvements in students' mental health literacy with use of a mental health curriculum in Canadian schools. *BioMed Cent.* **2014**, *14*, 379–385. [CrossRef] [PubMed]

90. Skre, I.; Friborg, O.; Breivik, C.; Johnsen, L.I.; Arnesen, Y.; Wang, C.E.A. A school intervention for mental health literacy in adolescents: Effects of a non-randomized cluster clinical trial. *BMC Public Health* **2013**, *13*, 873. [CrossRef] [PubMed]

91. Wahl, O.F.; Susin, J.; Kaplan, L.; Lax, A.; Zatina, D. Changing knowledge and attitudes with a middle school mental health education curriculum. *Stigma Res. Action* **2011**, *1*, 44–53. [CrossRef] [PubMed]

92. Watson, A.C.; Otey, E.; Westbook, A.L.; Gardner, A.L.; Lamb, T.A.; Corrigan, P.W.; Fenton, W.S. Changing middle schoolers' attitudes about mental illness through education. *Schizophr. Bull.* **2004**, *30*, 563–572. [CrossRef] [PubMed]

93. Jorm, A.E. Australian young people's awareness of Headspace, BeyondBlue and other mental health organizations. *Aust. Psychiatry* **2009**, *17*, 472–474. [CrossRef] [PubMed]

94. Fraser, E.; Pakenham, K.I. Resilience in children of parents with mental illness: Relations between mental health literacy, social connectedness and coping, and both adjustment and caregiving. *Psych. Health & Med.* **2009**, *14*, 573–584. [CrossRef]

95. Grové, C.; Reupert, A.E.; Maybery, D.J. The perspectives of young people of parents with a mental illness regarding preferred interventions and supports: "It's like a weight off your shoulders". *J. Child Family Stud.* **2016**, *25*, 3056–3065. [CrossRef]

96. Rickwood, D.; Cavanagh, S.; Curtis, L.; Sakrouge, R. Educating young people about mental health and mental illness: Evaluating a school-based programme. *Int. J. Ment. Health Promot.* **2004**, *6*, 23–32. [CrossRef]

97. Burns, J.R.; Rapee, R.M. Adolescent mental health literacy: Young people's knowledge of depression and help-seeking. *J. Adolesc.* **2006**, *29*, 225–229. [CrossRef] [PubMed]

98. Bosch, A.; Riebschleger, J.; van Loon, L. Dutch youth of parents with a mental illness reflect upon their feelings of guilt and shame. *Int. J. Ment. Health Promot.* **2017**, 1–14. [CrossRef]

99. Wright, A.; Harris, M.G.; Wiggers, J.H.; Jorm, A.F.; Cotton, S.M.; Harrigan, S.M.; McGorry, P.D. Recognition of depression and psychosis by young Australians and their beliefs about treatment. *Med. J. Aust.* **2005**, *183*, 143.

100. Lam, L.T. Mental health literacy and mental health status in adolescents: A population-bases survey. *Child Adolesc. Psychiatry Ment. Health* **2014**, *8*, 1–8. [CrossRef]

101. Henderson, P. Coping with mental illness: A program for middle school students. *Elem. School Guid. Couns.* **1993**, *27*, 198–208.

102. Riebschleger, J.; Onaga, E.; Tableman, B.; Bybee, D. Mental health consumer parents' recommendations for psychoeducation for their minor children. Special issue on parents with disability challenges. *Psychiatr. Rehabil. J.* **2014**, *37*, 183–185. [CrossRef] [PubMed]

103. Dam, K.; Hall, E.O.C. Navigating in an unpredictable daily life: A metasynthesis on children's experiences living with a parent with severe mental illness. *Scand. J. Caring Sci.* **2016**, *3*, 442–457. [CrossRef] [PubMed]

104. Serra, M.; Lai, A.; Puizza, C.; Pioli, R.; Preti, A.; Masala, C.; Petretto, D.R. Beliefs and attitudes among Italian high school students toward people with severe mood disorders. *J. Nerv. Disord.* **2013**, *201*, 311–318. [CrossRef] [PubMed]

105. Pinfold, V.; Toulmin, H.; Thornicroft, G.; Huxley, P.; Farmer, P.; Graham, T. Reducing psychiatric stigma and discrimination: Evaluation of educational interventions in UK secondary schools. *Br. J. Psychiatry* **2003**, *182*, 342–346. [CrossRef] [PubMed]

106. Bee, P.; Berzins, K.; Calam, R.; Pryjmachuk, S.; Abel, K.M. Defining quality of life in the children of parents with mental illness: A preliminary stakeholder-led model. *Early Interv. Psychiatry* **2013**, *7*, 109–122. [CrossRef] [PubMed]

107. Olsson, D.P.; Kennedy, M.G. Mental health literacy among young people in a small US town: Recognition of disorders and hypothetical helping responses. *Early Interv. Psychiatry* **2010**, *4*, 291–298. [CrossRef] [PubMed]

108. Yap, M.B.H.; Jorm, A.F. The influence of stigma on first aid actions by young people for mental health problems in a close friend or family member: Finding from an Australian national survey of youth. *J. Affect. Disord.* **2011**, *134*, 473–477. [CrossRef] [PubMed]

109. Jorm, A.F. Mental health literacy: Empowering the community to take action for better mental health. *Am. Psychol.* **2011**, *67*, 231–243. [CrossRef] [PubMed]

110. Bibou-Nakou, I. 'Troubles Talk' among professionals working with families facing parental mental illness. *J. Family Stud.* **2003**, *9*, 248–268. [CrossRef]

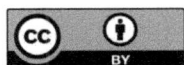

![brain sciences logo](brain sciences)

Concept Paper

Promoting Mental Health in Unaccompanied Refugee Minors: Recommendations for Primary Support Programs

Usama El-Awad *, Atefeh Fathi **, Franz Petermann and Tilman Reinelt**

Center for Clinical Psychology and Rehabilitation, University of Bremen, Grazer Str. 6, 28359 Bremen, Germany;
fathi@uni-bremen.de (A.F.); fpeterm@uni-bremen.de (F.P.); reinelt@uni-bremen.de (T.R.)
* Correspondence: elawad@uni-bremen.de; Tel.: +49-421-2186-8634

Received: 1 August 2017; Accepted: 18 October 2017; Published: 1 November 2017

Abstract: During the last years, the number of refugees around the world increased to about 22.5 million. The mental health of refugees, especially of unaccompanied minors (70% between the ages of 16 and 18 years) who have been exposed to traumatic events (e.g., war), is generally impaired with symptoms of post-traumatic stress disorder, depression, and anxiety. Several studies revealed (1) a huge variation among the prevalence rates of these mental problems, and (2) that post-migration stressors (e.g., language barriers, cultural differences) might be at least as detrimental to mental health as the traumatic events in pre- and peri-flight. As psychotherapy is a limited resource that should be reserved for severe cases and as language trainings are often publicly offered for refugees, we recommend focusing on intercultural competence, emotion regulation, and goal setting and goal striving in primary support programs: Intercultural competence fosters adaptation by giving knowledge about cultural differences in values and norms. Emotion regulation regarding empathy, positive reappraisal, and cultural differences in emotion expression fosters both adaptation and mental health. Finally, supporting unaccompanied refugee minors in their goal setting and goal striving is necessary, as they carry many unrealistic wishes and unattainable goals, which can be threatening to their mental health. Building on these three psychological processes, we provide recommendations for primary support programs for unaccompanied refugee minors that are aged 16 to 18 years.

Keywords: refugees; mental health; adaptation; acculturation; intercultural competence; emotion regulation; motivation

---

1. Introduction

Due to wars and disasters, the number of forcibly displaced people in 2016 increased to 65.6 million worldwide. These included 22.5 million refugees, of which 2.8 million were asylum seekers. Half of the refugees were underage and about 75,000 asylum applications were lodged by unaccompanied minors [1]. Germany received about half of these applications with 91.1% coming from male and 8.9% coming from female unaccompanied refugee minors (URM) [2]. More than 70% of all URM were between 16 and 18 years old [3]. Hence, supporting unaccompanied refugee minors (URM) is of importance to the German welfare and school system, especially for the youth welfare service as it assumes responsibility for URM by taking over the legal guardianship. The main function of the youth welfare service is to support children and adolescents in their development. However, in Germany, despite this responsibility and the large amount of refugees, there are no guidelines for programs that are research based, which target adaptation and mental health and cover different dimensions related to URM. Therefore, our aim is to introduce a framework that can guide practitioners in designing their programs. As several psychological research areas, e.g., clinical psychology, cultural psychology, and social psychology, contribute to the study of adaptation and mental health, the framework cannot rely on a coherent theory. Rather, it aims to represent the various research lines while drawing on cognitive, affective, and motivational concepts affecting mental health and adaptation, as these concepts are generally the focus of training (e.g., intercultural competence (IC), emotion regulation, goal setting and goal striving).

For many years, concerns focused on URM's well-being with regard to physical diseases and injuries that are caused by disasters and wars [4]. However, although many refugees endure physical injuries or hunger, far more suffer psychologically from traumatic experiences [5]. These experiences include, for instance, the experience of life-threatening events, physical maltreatment, sexual abuse, the loss of loved ones, separation from ones family against ones will, or the witnessing of violence towards others [6,7]. Especially, URM are at a higher risk of experiencing multiple traumatic events [7,8]. Hence, mental health problems, e.g., Post-Traumatic Stress Disorder (PTSD), Major Depression Disorder (MDD), Generalized Anxiety Disorder (GAD), Adjustive Disorders, Panic attacks and Somatization, have commonly been reported among URM [5,9–11]. However, the prevalence rates of diagnoses differ largely between studies, disorders, and types of measures. For instance, the prevalence rates of PTSD, as derived from self-reports on questionnaires, vary between 17% and 71%, while prevalence rates derived from clinical interviews vary between 20% and 30%. Similarly, prevalence rates for MDD vary between 9% in clinical interviews and 44% in self-reported questionnaires, while the prevalence rates for GAD vary between 4% in clinical interviews and 38% in self-report questionnaires. Hence, about 20% to 80% of URM show little psychopathological concerns and seem to be resilient [8]. In addition to being resilient from the beginning, the mental health of the majority of URM improves over time [12], thereby resembling the typical trajectories in adjustments to chronic stress or post traumatic events [13]. However, these positive adjustments might take some time as they have been reported in a 9-year follow-up study [12], while no improvements in the mental health of URM were observed within the first two years after their arrival in the host country [14,15].

2. Acculturation and Mental Heath

This high maintenance of mental health problems in URM during the first years after arrival might reflect post-migration stressors rather than the lasting impact of experienced traumatic events pre- or during the flight. Indeed, URM reported an increase in stressful life events within the first two years after arrival in the host country [14], which were mainly due to experiences of discrimination (e.g., feelings that others have prejudices about oneself or one's country), insufficient housing conditions, or a general dissatisfaction with one's leisure time [15,16]. In addition, there are cultural changes leading URM to the feeling of living in two different worlds [5]: People look different, wear a different wardrobe, speak a different language, eat different food, live by different religions, values, moral codes, or differ in their general way of thinking. According to Berry's influential framework [17,18], this situation leads to processes of acculturation, i.e., changes in the perception of one's own culture that take place due to contact with culturally dissimilar people or influences. Culture thereby refers to shared understandings or meanings kept by a specific group of people. The similarity between the host culture and the heritage culture determines the strength of the acculturation process during the adaption to the host culture [19]. If URM only need to learn some new aspects on how to deal within their host culture, the adaptation process will be rather smooth. However, if there are serious conflicts between appropriate behaviors in their heritage culture and in the host culture, or acculturation-specific daily hassles (e.g., perceived discrimination), this might result in acculturative stress [17,20], which usually manifests itself in mental disorders such as depression, anxiety, or in some cases in psychosis [21].

Indeed, URM reported an increased amount of both acculturation-specific and general hassles as compared to their peers from the host country and their peers with immigrant background but without flight experience [22,23]. Associations between daily hassles and symptoms of depression remained even after influences of traumatic events pre- or during the flight had been controlled [24,25].

In addition, longitudinal analyses revealed that the extent of acculturation-specific daily hassles predicted the trajectories in adaptation to traumatic events. A lower extent of daily hassles predicted resilient trajectories right from the beginning, while a higher extent of daily hassles predicted chronic trajectories as well as improved trajectories [26]. Furthermore, regarding the causal direction, these models supported an influence of daily hassles on depressive symptoms rather than an influence of depressive symptoms on daily hassles [26]. Hence, the elevated risk for daily hassles in URM cannot be explained by their traumatic experiences.

In addition to daily hassles, the amount of acculturative stress URM experience is influenced by their acculturation strategies [17,18]. Acculturation strategies are based on two components: (1) orientation (i.e., attitudes and activities) towards the host culture and (2) orientation towards the heritage culture. Based on these two orientations, four acculturation strategies can be derived: integration, assimilation, separation, and marginalization. Integration is defined by both an orientation towards the host culture and an orientation towards the heritage culture. In contrast, assimilation is denoted by an orientation towards the host culture, but no orientation towards the heritage culture, while separation is described by no orientation towards the host culture, but an orientation towards the heritage culture. Finally, marginalization is defined by both no orientation towards the host culture and no orientation towards the heritage culture [18]. Across several studies, integration has been regarded as the most favorable orientation in terms of acculturation and mental health. Adolescent refugees following an integrative orientation demonstrated a higher self-esteem, had more close friends, and were more accepted by their peers as compared to refugee adolescents following other acculturation strategies [27]. An integrative orientation was related to less depressed mood after controlling for traumatic experiences, however, no differences to an assimilation strategy were reported, whereas both separation and marginalization strategies were associated with an elevated depressive mood [25]. In addition, adolescent refugees applying a marginalization strategy were at a greater risk of experiencing daily hassles, indicating an interaction of acculturation strategies and post-migration stressors [25].

In addition, acculturation is a process that occurs over time. According to Berry [28], there are three distinguishable phases: contact with the host culture, conflict with the host culture, and adaptation to the host culture. Contact lies at the core of acculturation as the purpose, nature, duration, and permanence of contact affect the acculturation process. For instance, Berry [28] noted that if the contact with the host culture has no purpose and is rather random, then the contact will be short-termed. In particular, communication is remarkably important during the contact phase and needs to be constructive and without failures and misunderstandings as much as it is possible [28]. Therefore, sensitivity to cultural differences is a prerequisite for a successful intercultural communication and the basis for a more general intercultural competence [29].

3. Acculturation and Intercultural Competence

With significantly rising global diversity, intercultural competence (IC) is considered a significant aspect of acculturation, biculturalism, or multiculturalism [30]. It reflects the effectiveness of people's communication and their activities together [29]. Therefore, IC can be described as the capability to appropriately and effectively carry out social interactions and communicate with people from various cultures based on one's own intercultural knowledge, skills, and attitudes [31].

Kim [32], as the first one who examined the role of communication in the acculturation process, discussed that the communication environment is strongly linked to personal and social communication and can be considered as a significant determinant of acculturation. The frequency and intensity of interactions and communication with members of the host society has a remarkable influence on immigrants' acculturation process. Hence, communication in the first phase of acculturation, when contacts to the host society are established, is crucial [33]. While involvement in their native ethnic community may foster the acculturation process of URM in the beginning, it may delay the acculturation process in the long-term. This is because the acculturation process mostly adopts and adapts to focal patterns and rules of communication in the host society. Moreover, the immigrants' communication competence can facilitate all of the other aspects of adaptation and adjustment in the host culture, so that intercultural communication competence can be considered as both the fundamental process and the main outcome of the acculturation process [34]. During the acculturation process, IC develops from an unconscious incompetence to an unconscious competence [35], as sensitivity to cultural differences grows and, thereby, shapes the competence for intercultural communication [29].

Among other factors that affect the levels of IC, emotion regulation might be particularly important as especially empathy may enable URM to reach a level of unconscious competence behavior and adapt to intercultural differences [36,37] while emotion dysregulation has been shown to be detrimental for IC [38]. In addition, competencies in emotion regulation have been associated with better mental health in general.

4. Emotion Regulation and Mental Health

Emotion regulation can be described as a process of the person's capability to evaluate, manage, experience, express and improve emotional reactions in a way that helps proper functioning [39]. It leads to a higher ability to appropriately respond to emotional experiences and can be seen as a dynamic process in which positive and negative emotions are being increased or decreased by using emotion regulation strategies [39,40]. Within Gross' [39] Process Modell of Emotion Regulation, strategies are categorized by the time they first affect the process in which emotions are being unfolded. Antecedent-focused strategies differ from response-focused strategies and precede physiological or behavioral responding on emotions. These include the reappraisal strategy, which is leading to most positive outcomes by changing the way in which a situation is interpreted and decreasing its emotional impact [41]. It changes cognition by deciding on alternative meanings of previously selected situational aspects [39].

Emotion regulation strategies both facilitate the acculturation process and are generally helpful to deal with traumatic experiences [42]. For instance, there are experimental evidences that the execution of adaptive emotion regulation strategies such as reappraisal can significantly diminish rage and aggression [43,44]. In contrast, emotion dysregulation has been associated with impaired anger management [45–48].

Regarding refugees, they not only experience extreme fear or shame because of traumatic experiences, but also often have difficulties with emotion regulation and anger management [49,50]. In addition, in a study on formerly abducted adolescents, who had been living in Ugandese rebel camps, difficulties in emotion regulation were associated with exacerbated symptoms of PTSD or depression [51] and emotion dysregulation mediated the effects of traumatic experiences on symptoms of PTSD, depression, and anger [52]. An additional study on the relation of emotion dysregulation, post-migration living difficulties and PTSD revealed a partial mediation of the effects of post-migration living difficulties on symptoms of PTSD and depression through emotion dysregulation, as well as a complete mediation of the effects of post-migration living difficulties on anger [52]. Consequently, impaired emotion regulation might act as a mechanism empowering the connection between asylum seekers and refugees' experiences and mental health outcomes [52]. The experience of extreme emotional distress in connection with trauma and post-migration living difficulties might force the refugees to use dysfunctional emotion regulation strategies and the lack of access to functional strategies may thus empower the association between post-migration living difficulties and PTSD and depression symptoms [52].

5. Goal Setting and Goal Striving and Mental Health

In addition to emotion dysregulation, post-migration living difficulties and the experience of traumatic events in refugees have been associated with difficulties in engaging in goal-directed behavior [52]. Upon their arrival in a host country URM have expectations towards the new country and goals that they like to achieve. They might expect living in peace, getting a good education, finding a well-paid job, or living in nice houses. However, finding a nice house is not always easy. It takes some time to get a place in a school or vocational school; educational degrees from home countries are not always accepted, and getting a well-paid job is rather difficult and sometimes impossible [53–55]. Thus, not all expectations or goals of URM can be met. Problems to disengage from unattainable goals, however, have been associated with depressive symptoms and a poorer mental health in general [56–58]. Indeed, unmet expectations regarding the host country have been reported both by clinicians treating Somali refugees in the United Kingdom and the USA [59] as well as Sudanese refugees in Canada [60] and have been related to psychological problems [60].

Several motivational strategies have been developed in order to help people setting attainable goals and striving for them. For instance, the strategy of mental contrasting (MC) connects people's wishes with obstacles impeding their fulfillment [61]. During MC people name a wish and elaborate on it through imagining in detail the best possible outcomes associated with its attainment. Subsequently, people name an aspect of the reality, which hinders them in attaining their wish, and elaborate on it. This procedure leads people to align their wishes with their expectations of success. If expectations to accomplish one's wish are high, people view the aspect of reality as an obstacle and form a strong association between the positive outcome and this obstacle, which leads to an enhanced goal commitment, energization, and goal striving. However, if expectations to accomplish one's wish are low, people do not regard the impeding reality as an obstacle, no associations between the impeding reality and the positive outcomes are formed, and, consequently, goal commitment, energization, and goal striving are reduced [61–63]. Thus, MC leads to strengthened goal striving in the light of high expectations of success, but to weakened goal striving and goal disengagement in the light of low expectations of success. To further enhance goal striving for feasible goals, MC has often been combined with implementation intentions [64]. Implementation intentions are a specific form of plan in the form: If situations X occurs (when and where), I will perform behavior Y.

6. Programs Supporting URM's Mental Health and Adaptation

Despite the high number of resilient URM and factors influencing mental health other than pre-flight traumatic experiences, most clinical interventions addressing mental health of URM focus on PTSD [65]. However, therapeutical interventions in face-to-face settings are a limited resource and the need of cultural-sensitive translators for specific languages [66] further depletes the resource. Hence, psychotherapy should be reserved for severe cases, while support programs should also target other factors that are directly influencing mental health (e.g., emotion regulation strategies or strategies for goal setting and goal striving) as well as factors indirectly affecting mental health through the acculturation processes, e.g., intercultural competence [67].

In contrast, governmental or organizational programs mainly support acculturation processes. However, most programs focus on structural economic, educational, or health aspects, as for instance providing refugees with housing, schooling, or vocational education, or integration in the labor market [53–55,68]. One major prerequisite for integration in schools and especially in the labor market is language. Therefore, language courses are often offered by the public or non-profit organizations [69,70]. In addition, several states like Germany offer government-funded integration courses, which cover topics as the German legal system, history, important values of the society, as well as rights and obligations of residents and are sometimes directed at specific target groups as young adults or women [70].

However, these integration courses are generally only loosely based on psychological concepts that are known to influence acculturation (e.g., intercultural competence) and mental health. In addition, they often consider refugees as helpless individuals, who are not able to take care of their lives independently. Yet, on the contrary, refugees are mostly individuals with a strong intention to survive and pull through, who have come to the host country with their own wishes and goals [71]. In addition, while clinical programs tend to focus only on psychotherapy, integration courses ignore the mental health condition of refugees, and especially URM, at all.

Therefore, primary support programs, which are designed for groups of URM, should include both elements that directly aim to reduce sub-threshold psychopathologies as well as foster acculturation by integrating the URMs own goals.

7. A Working Model for Developing Primary Support Programs for Adaptation and Mental Health of URM

The reviewed literature on mental health and acculturation in URM revealed several key constructs—intercultural competence, emotion regulation, goal setting, and goal striving—that root in different lines of psychological research. While intercultural competence is mainly discussed in cultural and organizational psychology, emotion regulation is a key construct in clinical psychology and developmental psychopathology, whereas goal setting and goal striving are primarily rooted in social and motivational psychology. Consequently, so far, no unifying framework exists that could guide the development of primary support programs for URM. Figure 1, therefore, depicts a working model how such a framework could look like. As intercultural competence rather draws on cognitive processes, while emotion regulation, as well as goal setting and goal striving reflect affective or motivational processes, respectively, the three processes might constitute rather independent ways to influence adaptation and mental health. However, in order to develop primary support programs for URM it would be critical that these three concepts—IC, emotion regulation, goal setting and goal striving—could actually be trained within the age of 16–18 years, the main age group of URM [3].

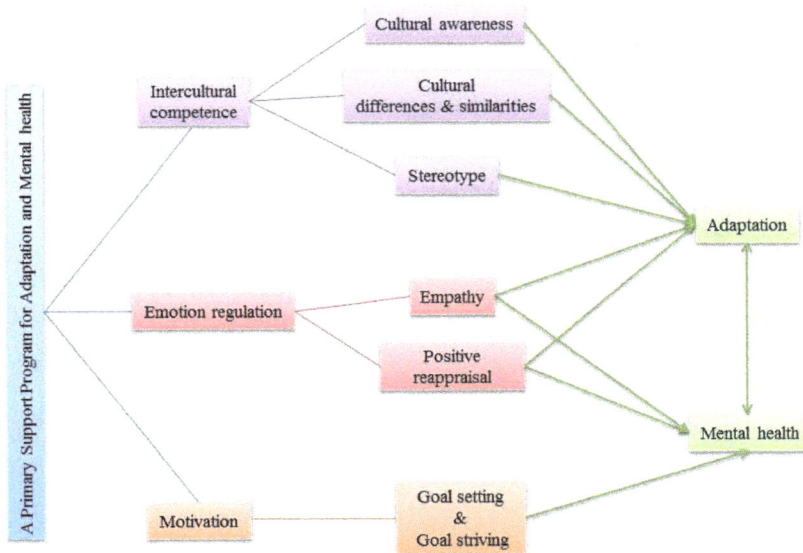

Figure 1. A working model for a primary support program for adaptation and mental health. A primary support program for unaccompanied refugee minors (URM) should include three main psychological elements: intercultural competence, emotion regulation and motivation. Training intercultural competence should include lessons on cultural awareness, cultural differences and similarities, and stereotypes in order to foster adaptation. Training emotion regulation should work on participant's empathy and strategies of emotional acceptance and emotional modification. This should foster the adaptation of URM and their mental health. During the motivation training, URM learn to set realistic goals and to strive for them efficiently, leading to improvements in mental health.

7.1. Training Intercultural Competence

As sensitivity to cultural differences is the basis for successful intercultural communication and IC in general [29], trainings of intercultural competence should include lessons on the concept of culture, cultural differences and similarities, stereotypes, adaptation skills, attitudes of respect and appreciation, and intercultural communication abilities. For instance, by giving knowledge about culture, URM will become more familiar with the norms, customs, cultural and social activities, the way of communicating and greeting, or the way of making friends in a host culture. Learning about cultural differences and similarities between refugees' heritage culture and a host culture, enables URM to balance their own cultural values and the host society's cultural values. In addition, learning about stereotypes that are related to different cultures, ethnicities and religions should help URM to understand other people's reactions and behaviors by informing them how stereotypes can affect people's reactions and expectations. Several training programs for IC have been developed for immigrants supporting a general effectiveness [72–74]. Hence, primary support programs for URM should include elements of IC.

7.2. Training Emotion Regulation

Based on Gross' model for emotion regulation [39], improving emotion regulation leads to a higher ability to appropriately respond to emotional experiences. It is especially empathy that is strongly linked to emotional competence [75], but training programs also focus on other strategies, as for instance on the acceptance of one's own emotions or reappraisal. Several studies revealed positive effects of emotion regulation trainings as part of a trauma-focused cognitive behavioral therapy, improving clinical outcomes and reducing dropout rates [76,77]. Similar effects have been reported for patients with major depression [76], as well as for non-clinical children and young adolescents [78]. With regard to refugees, studies on Cambodian refugees performing culturally adapted forms of cognitive behavioral therapy [79] suggested that progression in emotion regulation ability successfully accelerates PTSD symptom reduction [80]. In particular, emotion regulation strategies of acceptance and mindfulness were beneficial [38].

Hence, as emotion regulation capabilities are generally reduced in refugees and better emotion regulation strategies foster mental health and the acculturation process, primary support programs for URM should include elements of emotion regulation.

7.3. Training Goal Setting and Goal Striving

Mental contrasting is a common strategy of goal setting and has been successfully applied to various wishes (interpersonal concerns, health, academic performance) and populations, including depressive patients [81] and children with externalizing disorders [82]. In addition, with regard to goal striving, II are one of the most successful strategies to initiate behaviour. They are common in health psychology [83], have even been utilized by children with externalizing problems [84,85], and meta-analytical effects are moderate to high [86,87]. Effects are especially high, when MC and II are combined [88]. However, most studies investigated the effects of MC, II, and MCII with regard to goal attainment and only few evidence has been reported for effects of II on goal disengagement [89].

Hence, as URM often carry unrealistic expectancies and wishes towards their life in the host country, primary support programs for URM should help them in setting realistic goals, disengage from unattainable or unrealistic wishes, and strive efficiently towards goal attainment. The strategies of MC and II might be suited for support programs for URM, in particular, as they have proven their value for different populations and goals, including children and adolescents, as well as people suffering from internalizing and externalizing problems. In addition, the strategies are easy to administer and learn.

8. Discussion, Limitations and Recommendations for Practice and Research

Unaccompanied refugee minors are at a special risk for mental health problems due to traumatic experiences pre or during their flight as well as difficulties in the acculturation process. So far, support programs for URM either mainly focus on their traumatic experiences and resulting PTSD or on structural aspects as language and integration courses, integration into the schooling system or the labor market. However, these programs do not directly address psychological processes, which might offer URM resources, they might be able to use subsequently during their acculturation process. Primary support programs, which include elements of IC, emotion regulation, and goal setting and goal striving, therefore fill a gap. These elements are easy to integrate into the existing programs and can be applied in group settings, thereby reducing costs in terms of time or money. However, training material will need to be translated into the different languages of the URM currently coming into the host countries and validation studies should be carried out to ensure the material is culturally appropriate. Moreover, for larger groups it might be advisable to use translators and interpreters, who are more familiar with the refugees' cultural backgrounds and have some experiences related to trainings or psychotherapies for refugees [66]. Due to the absence of a naturally-arising social support for URM, it is recommended to apply support programs, which connect them to the members of their own cultures and ethnicities. Such programs will help URM to receive social supports from both original and new cultures and subsequently reduce psychological difficulties [90].

While about 70% of the URM are between 16 and 18 years [3], it is unclear whether primary support programs for younger URM can rely on all three concepts. Both emotion regulation trainings and II have been successfully applied to children aged 9 to 12 years [78,84], however little is known on trainings of IC in this age group and none of concepts has generally been trained in even younger children. Hence, the appropriateness of training these concepts in younger children remains a question of future research.

In addition, longitudinal studies are needed in order to evaluate the effectiveness of these program elements and whether the elements affect adaptation and mental health independently of each other or are interrelated. Furthermore, future research needs to analyze the personal characteristics of URM or the program conductors, which might act as potential moderators for the success of primary support programs. Finally, the three described elements influencing mental health and adaptation are not exclusive and other constructs should be evaluated with regard to trainability and their supporting effects.

Conflicts of Interest: The authors declare no conflict of interest.

References

1. UNHCR. Global Trends: Forced Displacement in 2017. Available online: http://www.unhcr.org/statistics/unhcrstats/5943e8a34/global-trends-forced-displacement-2016.html (accessed on 24 July 2017).
2. Bundesamt Für Migration und Flüchtlinge. Aktuelle Zahlen zu Asyl. Den Menschen im Blick. Schützen. Integrieren 2016. Available online: https://www.bamf.de/SharedDocs/Anlagen/DE/Publikationen/Broschueren/ (accessed on 11 October 2017).
3. Arbeitsgemeinschaft für Kinder- und Jugendhilfe. Unbegleitete Minderjährige Flüchtlinge—Bedingungen für Nachhaltige Integration Schaffen Positionspapier der Arbeitsgemeinschaft für Kinder- und Jugendhilfe—AGJ 2016. Available online: https://www.agj.de/fileadmin/files/positionen/2016/Positionspapier_Unbegleitete_minderj%C3%A4hrige_Fl%C3%BCchtlinge.pdf (accessed on 11 October 2017).
4. Birman, D.; Beehler, S.; Harris, E.; Everson, M.L.; Batia, K.; Liautaud, J.; Frazier, S.; Atkins, M.; Blanton, S.; Buwalda, J.; et al. International family, adult, and child enhancement services (FACES): A community-based comprehensive services model for refugee children in resettlement. *Am. J. Orthopsychiatry* **2008**, *78*, 121–132. [CrossRef] [PubMed]

5. Carswell, K.; Blackburn, P.; Barker, C. The relationship between trauma, post-migration problems and the psychological well-being of refugees and asylum seekers. *Int. J. Soc. Psychiatry* **2011**, *57*, 107–119. [CrossRef] [PubMed]

6. Bean, T.; Derluyn, I.; Eurelings-Bontekoe, E.; Broekaert, E.; Spinhoven, P. Comparing psychological distress, traumatic stress reactions, and experiences of unaccompanied refugee minors with experiences of adolescents accompanied by parents. *J. Nerv. Ment. Dis.* **2007**, *195*, 288–297. [CrossRef] [PubMed]

7. Derluyn, I.; Mels, C.; Broekaert, E. Mental health problems in separated refugee adolescents. *J. Adolesc. Health* **2009**, *44*, 291–297. [CrossRef] [PubMed]

8. Witt, A.; Rassenhofer, M.; Fegert, J.M.; Plener, P.L. Demand for help and provision of services in the care of unaccompanied refugee minors. A systematic review. *Kindh. Entwickl.* **2015**, *24*, 209–224. [CrossRef]

9. Bronstein, I.; Montgomery, P.; Dobrowolski, S. PTSD in asylum-seeking male adolescents from Afghanistan. *J. Trauma. Stress* **2012**, *25*, 551–557. [CrossRef] [PubMed]

10. Vervliet, M.; Demott, M.A.M.; Jakobsen, M.; Broekaert, E.; Heir, T.; Derluyn, I. The mental health of unaccompanied refugee minors on arrival in the host country. *Scand. J. Psychol.* **2014**, *55*, 33–37. [CrossRef] [PubMed]

11. Petermann, F.; Petermann, U. Refugee Minors. *Kindh. Entwickl.* **2016**, *25*, 201–203. [CrossRef]

12. Montgomery, E. Trauma and resilience in young refugees: A 9-year follow-up study. *Dev. Psychopathol.* **2010**, *22*, 477–489. [CrossRef] [PubMed]

13. Bonanno, G.A.; Diminich, E.D. Annual Research Review: Positive adjustment to adversity—Trajectories of minimal-impact resilience and emergent resilience. *J. Child Psychol. Psychiatry* **2013**, *54*, 378–401. [CrossRef] [PubMed]

14. Jensen, T.K.; Skardalsmo, E.M.B.; Fjermestad, K.W. Development of mental health problems—A follow-up study of unaccompanied refugee minors. *Child Adolesc. Psychiatry Ment. Health* **2014**, *8*, 29. [CrossRef] [PubMed]

15. Vervliet, M.; Lammertyn, J.; Broekaert, E.; Derluyn, I. Longitudinal follow-up of the mental health of unaccompanied refugee minors. *Eur. Child Adolesc. Psychiatry.* **2014**, *23*, 337–346. [CrossRef] [PubMed]

16. Edge, S.; Newbold, B. Discrimination and the health of immigrants and refugees: Exploring Canada's evidence base and directions for future research in newcomer receiving countries. *J. Immigr. Minor. Health* **2013**, *15*, 141–148. [CrossRef] [PubMed]

17. Berry, J.W. Immigration, acculturation and adaptation. *Appl. Psychol.* **1997**, *46*, 5–68. [CrossRef]

18. Berry, J.W. Acculturation: Living successfully in two cultures. *Int. J. Intercult. Relat.* **2005**, *29*, 697–712. [CrossRef]

19. Rudmin, F.W. Critical History of the Acculturation Psychology of Assimilation, Separation, Integration, and Marginalization. *Rev. Gen. Psychol.* **2003**, *7*, 3–37. [CrossRef]

20. *Cambridge Handbook of Acculturation Psychology*; Sam, D.L.; Berry, J.W. (Eds.) Cambridge University Press: Cambridge, UK, 2006.

21. Renner, W.; Berry, J.W. The ineffectiveness of group interventions for female Turkish migrants with recurrent depression. *J. Soc. Behav. Personal.* **2011**, *39*, 1217–1234. [CrossRef]

22. Keles, S.; Friborg, O.; Idsoe, T.; Sirin, S.; Oppedal, B. Resilience and acculturation among unaccompanied refugee minors. *Int. J. Behav. Dev.* **2016**. [CrossRef]

23. Seglem, K.B.; Oppedal, B.; Roysamb, E. Daily hassles and coping dispositions as predictors of psychological adjustment. A comparative study of young unaccompanied refugees and youth in the resettlement country. *Int. J. Behav. Dev.* **2014**, *38*, 293–303. [CrossRef]

24. Keles, S.; Friborg, O.; Idsoe, T.; Sirin, S.; Oppedal, B. Depression among unaccompanied minor refugees: The relative contribution of general and acculturation-specific daily hassles. *Ethn. Health* **2016**, *21*, 300–317. [CrossRef] [PubMed]

25. Lincoln, A.K.; Lazarevic, V.; White, M.T.; Ellis, B.H. The impact of acculturation style and acculturative hassles on the mental health of Somali adolescent refugees. *J. Immigr. Minor. Health* **2016**, *18*, 771–778. [CrossRef] [PubMed]

26. Keles, S.; Idsoe, T.; Friborg, O.; Sirin, S.; Oppedal, B. The longitudinal relation between daily hassles and depressive symptoms among unaccompanied refugees in Norway. *J. Abnorm. Child Psychol.* **2016**. [CrossRef] [PubMed]

27. Kovacev, L.; Shute, R. Acculturation and social support in relation to psychosocial adjustment of adolescent refugees re-settled in Australia. *Int. J. Behav. Dev.* **2004**, *28*, 259–267. [CrossRef]
28. Berry, J.W. Acculturation as Varieties of Adaptation. In *Acculturation: Theory, Models and Findings*; Padilla, A., Ed.; Westview: Boulder, CO, USA, 1980.
29. Hammer, M.R.; Bennett, M.J.; Wiseman, R. Measuring intercultural sensitivity: The intercultural development inventory. *Int. J. Intercult. Relat.* **2003**, *27*, 421–443. [CrossRef]
30. Arasaratnam, L.A.; Doerfel, M.L. Intercultural communication competence: Identifying key components from multicultural perspectives. *Int. J. Intercult. Relat.* **2005**, *29*, 137–163. [CrossRef]
31. Deardorff, D.K. The identification and assessment of intercultural competence as a student outcome of internationalization at institutions of higher education in the United States. *J. Stud. Int. Educ.* **2006**, *10*, 241–266. [CrossRef]
32. Kim, Y.Y. *Communication and Cross-Cultural Adaptation: An Integrative Theory*; Multilingual Matters: Clevedon, UK, 1988.
33. Kajiura, A. Analysis of previous researches on intercultural communication. *Polyglossia* **2007**, *13*, 59–68.
34. Arasaratnam, L.A. The development of a new instrument of intercultural communication competence. *J. Intercult. Commun.* **2009**, *20*, 1404–1634.
35. Cannon, H.M.; Feinstein, A.F.; Friesen, D.P. Managing complexity: Applying the conscious-competence model to experiential learning. *Dev. Bus. Simul. Exp. Learn.* **2010**, *37*, 172–182.
36. Bennett, M.J. Becoming interculturally competent. In *Toward Multiculturalism: A Reader in Multicultural Education*; Intercultural Resource Corporation: Newton, MA, USA, 2004.
37. Herfst, S.L.; van Oudenhoven, J.P.; Timmerman, M.E. Intercultural Effectiveness Training in three Western immigrant countries: A cross-cultural evaluation of critical incident. *Int. J. Intercult. Relat.* **2008**, *32*, 67–80. [CrossRef]
38. Hinton, D.E.; Nickerson, A.; Bryant, R.A. Worry, worry attacks, and PTSD among Cambodian refugees: A path analysis investigation. *Soc. Sci. Med.* **2011**, *72*, 1817–1825. [CrossRef] [PubMed]
39. Gross, J.J. Emotion regulation: Affective, cognitive, and social consequences. *Psychophysiology* **2002**, *39*, 281–291. [CrossRef] [PubMed]
40. Parrott, W.G. Beyond hedonism: Motives for inhibiting good moods and for maintaining bad moods. In *Handbook of Mental Control*; Wegner, D.M., Penebaker, J.W., Eds.; Prentice Hall: Englewood Cliffs, NJ, USA, 1993; pp. 278–308.
41. Gross, J.J.; John, O.P. Individual differences in two emotion regulation processes: Implications for affect, relationships, and well-being. *J. Personal. Soc. Psychol.* **2003**, *85*, 348–362. [CrossRef]
42. Seligowski, A.V.; Lee, D.J.; Bardeen, J.R.; Orcutt, H.K. Emotion regulation and posttraumatic stress symptoms: A meta-analysis. *Cogn. Behav. Ther.* **2015**, *44*, 87–102. [CrossRef] [PubMed]
43. Denson, T.F.; Moulds, M.L.; Grisham, J.R. The effects of analytical rumination, reappraisal, and distraction on anger experience. *Behav. Ther.* **2012**, *43*, 355–364. [CrossRef] [PubMed]
44. Szasz, P.L.; Szentagotai, A.; Hofmann, S.G. The effect of emotion regulation strategies on anger. *Behav. Res. Ther.* **2011**, *49*, 114–119. [CrossRef] [PubMed]
45. Besharat, M.A.; Nia, M.E.; Farahani, H. Anger and major depressive disorder: The mediating role of emotion regulation and anger rumination. *Asian J. Psychiatry* **2013**, *6*, 35–41. [CrossRef] [PubMed]
46. Mauss, I.B.; Cook, C.L.; Cheng, J.Y.; Gross, J.J. Individual differences in cognitive reappraisal: Experiential and physiological responses to an anger provocation. *Int. J. Psychophysiol.* **2007**, *66*, 116–124. [CrossRef] [PubMed]
47. Memedovic, S.; Grisham, J.R.; Denson, T.F.; Molds, M.L. The effects of trait reappraisal and suppression on anger and blood pressure in response to provocation. *J. Res. Personal.* **2010**, *44*, 540–543. [CrossRef]
48. Shorey, R.C.; Cornelius, T.L.; Idema, C. Trait anger as a mediator of difficulties with emotion regulation and female-perpetrated psychological aggression. *Violence Vict.* **2011**, *26*, 271–282. [CrossRef] [PubMed]
49. Fazel, M.; Wheeler, J.; Danesh, J. Prevalence of serious mental disorder in 7000 refugees resettled in western countries: A systematic review. *Lancet* **2005**, *365*, 1309–1314. [CrossRef]
50. Steel, Z.; Chey, T.; Silove, D.; Marnane, C.; Bryant, R.A.; van Ommeren, M. Association of torture and other potentially traumatic events with mental health outcomes among populations exposed to mass conflict and displacement: A systematic review and meta-analysis. *J. Am. Med. Assoc.* **2009**, *302*, 537–549. [CrossRef] [PubMed]

51. Amone-P'Olak, K.; Garnefski, N.; Kraaij, V. Adolescents caught between fires: Cognitive emotion regulation in response to war experiences in Northern Uganda. *J. Adolesc.* **2007**, *30*, 655–669. [CrossRef] [PubMed]
52. Nickerson, A.; Bryant, R.A.; Silove, D.; Steel, Z. A critical review of psychological treatments of posttraumatic stress disorder in refugees. *Clin. Psychol. Rev.* **2011**, *31*, 399–417. [CrossRef] [PubMed]
53. Schroeder, J.; Seukwa, L.H. Access to education in Germany. In *Structural Context of Refugee Integration in Canada and Germany*; Korntheuer, A., Pritchard, P., Maehler, D.B., Eds.; GESIS Series (15); GESIS—Leibniz Institute for the Social Sciences: Cologne, Germany, 2017.
54. Sherell, K. Access to housing in Canada. In *Structural Context of Refugee Integration in Canada and Germany*; Korntheuer, A., Pritchard, P., Maehler, D.B., Eds.; GESIS Series (15); GESIS—Leibniz Institute for the Social Sciences: Cologne, Germany, 2017.
55. Wilkinson, L. The labour market experiences of refugees in Canada. In *Structural Context of Refugee Integration in Canada and Germany*; Korntheuer, A., Pritchard, P., Maehler, D.B., Eds.; GESIS Series (15); GESIS—Leibniz Institute for the Social Sciences: Cologne, Germany, 2017.
56. Klinger, E. Consequences of commitment to and disengagement from incentives. *Psychol. Rev.* **1975**, *82*, 1–25. [CrossRef]
57. Kraaij, V.; Garnefski, N. Cognitive, behavioral and goal adjustment coping and depressive symptoms in young people with diabetes: A search for intervention targets for coping skills training. *J. Clin. Psychol. Med. Settings* **2015**, *22*, 45–53. [CrossRef] [PubMed]
58. Wrosch, C.; Scheier, M.F.; Carver, C.S.; Schulz, R. The importance of goal disengagement in adaptive self-regulation: When giving up is beneficial. *Self Identity* **2003**, *2*, 1–20. [CrossRef]
59. Warfa, N.; Curtis, S.; Watters, C.; Carswell, K.; Ingleby, D.; Bhui, K. Migration experiences, employment status and psychological distress among Somali immigrants: A mixed-method international study. *BMC Public Health* **2012**, *12*, 749. [CrossRef] [PubMed]
60. Simich, L.; Hamilton, H.; Khamisa Baya, B. Mental Distress, Economic Hardship and Expectations of Life in Canada among Sudanese Newcomers. *Transcult. Psychiatry* **2006**, *43*, 418–444. [CrossRef] [PubMed]
61. Oettingen, G. Future thought and behavioral change. *Eur. Rev. Soc. Psychol.* **2012**, *23*, 1–63. [CrossRef]
62. Kappes, A.; Oettingen, G. The emergence of goal pursuit: Mental contrasting connects future and reality. *J. Exp. Soc. Psychol.* **2014**, *54*, 25–39. [CrossRef]
63. Kappes, A.; Wendt, M.; Reinelt, T.; Oettingen, G. Mental contrasting changes the meaning of reality. *J. Exp. Soc. Psychol.* **2013**, *49*, 797–810. [CrossRef]
64. Gollwitzer, P.M. Implementation intentions: Strong effects of simple plans. *Am. Psychol.* **1999**, *54*, 493–503. [CrossRef]
65. Anders, M.; Christiansen, H. Unaccompanied refugee minors: A systematic review of psychological interventions. *Kindh. Entwickl.* **2016**, *25*, 216–230. [CrossRef]
66. Björn, G.J. Ethics and interpreting in psychotherapy with refugee children and families. *Nord. J. Psychiatry* **2005**, *59*, 516–521. [CrossRef] [PubMed]
67. Reinelt, T.; Vasileva, M.; Petermann, F. Refugee children's mental health problems: Beyond posttraumatic stress disorder. *Kindh. Entwickl.* **2016**, *25*, 231–237. [CrossRef]
68. Valenta, M.; Bunar, N. State assisted integration: Refugee integration policies in Scandinavian welfare states: The Swedish and Norwegian experience. *J. Refug. Stud.* **2010**, *23*, 463–483. [CrossRef]
69. Atallah, N. Access to resettlement services in Canada. In *Structural Context of Refugee Integration in Canada and Germany*; GESIS Series (15); Korntheuer, A., Pritchard, P., Maehler, D.B., Eds.; GESIS—Leibniz Institute for the Social Sciences: Cologne, Germany, 2017.
70. Prem, M. Access to resettlement services in Germany: Language options for refugees and asylum seekers in Germany. In *Structural Context of Refugee Integration in Canada and Germany*; Korntheuer, A., Pritchard, P., Maehler, D.B., Eds.; GESIS Series (15); GESIS—Leibniz Institute for the Social Sciences: Cologne, Germany, 2017.
71. Murray, K.; Davidson, G.; Schweitzer, R. Review of refugee mental health interventions following resettlement: Best practices and recommendations. *Am. J. Orthopsychiatry* **2010**, *80*, 576–585. [CrossRef] [PubMed]
72. Bhawuk, D.; Brislin, R. Cross-cultural Training: A Review. *Appl. Psychol.* **2000**, *49*, 162–191. [CrossRef]
73. Black, J.S.; Mendenhall, M. Cross-Cultural Training Effectiveness: A Review and a Theoretical Framework for Future Research. *Acad. Manag. Rev.* **2009**, *15*, 113–136.

74. Montalvo, F.F.; Lasater, T.T.; Valdez, N.G. Training child welfare workers for cultural awareness: the culture simulator technique. *Child Welfare* **1982**, *61*, 341–352. [PubMed]

75. Saarni, C. Children's emotional-expressive behaviors as regulators of others' happy and sad states. *New Dir. Child Dev.* **2009**, *55*, 91–106. [CrossRef]

76. Berking, M.; Wupperman, P.; Reichardt, A.; Pejic, T.; Dippel, A.; Znoj, H. Emotion-regulation skills as a treatment target in psychotherapy. *Behav. Res. Ther. J.* **2008**, *46*, 1230–1237. [CrossRef] [PubMed]

77. Bryant, J.; McDonald, V.M.; Boyes, A.; Sanson-Fisher, R.; Paul, C.; Melville, J. Improving medication adherence in chronic obstructive pulmonary disease: A systematic review. *Respir. Res.* **2013**, *14*, 109–120. [CrossRef] [PubMed]

78. Von Marees, N.; Petermann, F. Förderung sozial-emotionaler Kompetenzen im Grundschulalter. *Kindh. Entwickl.* **2009**, *18*, 244–253.

79. Hinton, D.E.; Rivera, E.I.; Hofmann, S.G.; Barlow, D.H.; Otto, M.W. Adapting CBT for traumatized refugees and ethnic minority patients: Examples from culturally adapted CBT (CA-CBT). *Transcult. Psychiatry* **2012**, *49*, 340–365. [CrossRef] [PubMed]

80. Hinton, D.E.; Pich, V.; Hofmann, S.G.; Otto, M.W. Acceptance and Mindfulness Techniques as Applied to Refugee and Ethnic Minority Populations With PTSD: Examples From "Culturally Adapted CBT". *Cogn. Behav. Pract.* **2013**, *20*, 33–46. [CrossRef]

81. Fritzsche, A.; Schlier, B.; Oettingen, G.; Lincoln, T.M. Mental Contrasting with Implementation Intentions Increases Goal-Attainment in Individuals with Mild to Moderate Depression. *Cogn. Ther. Res.* **2016**, *40*, 557–564. [CrossRef]

82. Gawrilow, C.; Morgenroth, K.; Schultz, R.; Oettingen, G.; Gollwitzer, P. Mental contrasting with implementation intentions enhances self-regulation of goal pursuit in schoolchildren at risk for ADHD. *Motiv. Emot.* **2013**, *37*, 134–145. [CrossRef]

83. Hagger, M.S.; Chatzisarantis, N.L.D.; Alberts, H.; Anggono, C.O.; Batailler, C.; Birt, A.R.; Brand, R.; Brandt, M.J.; Brewer, G.; Bruyneel, S.; et al. A Multilab Preregistered Replication of the Ego-Depletion Effect. *Perspect. Psychol. Sci.* **2016**, *11*, 546–573. [CrossRef] [PubMed]

84. Gawrilow, C.; Gollwitzer, P.M. Implementation intentions facilitate response inhibition in children with ADHD. *Cogn. Ther. Res.* **2008**, *32*, 261–280. [CrossRef]

85. Guderjahn, L.; Gold, A.; Stadler, G.; Gawrilow, C. Self-regulation strategies support children with ADHD to overcome symptom-related behavior in the classroom. *Atten. Deficit Hyperact. Disord.* **2013**, *5*, 397–407. [CrossRef] [PubMed]

86. Adriaanse, M.A.; Vinkers, C.D.; De Ridder, D.T.; Hox, J.J.; De Wit, J.B. Do implementation intentions help to eat a healthy diet? A systematic review and meta-analysis of the empirical evidence. *Appetite* **2011**, *56*, 183–193. [CrossRef] [PubMed]

87. Gollwitzer, P.M.; Sheeran, P. Implementation Intentions and Goal Achievement: A Meta-analysis of Effects and Processes. *Adv. Exp. Soc. Psychol.* **2006**, *38*, 69–119.

88. Oettingen, G.; Gollwitzer, P.M. Strategies of setting and implementing goals: Mental contrasting and implementation intentions. In *Social Psychological Foundations of Clinical Psychology*; Maddux, J.E., Tangney, J.P., Eds.; Guilford Press: New York, NY, USA, 2010; pp. 114–135.

89. Henderson, M.; Gollwitzer, P.M.; Oettingen, G. Implementation Intentions and Disengagement from a Failing Course of Action. *J. Behav. Decis. Mak.* **2007**, *20*, 81–102. [CrossRef]

90. Yasin, M.; Safree, M.A.; Adawiah, D.M. The relationship between social supports and psychological problems among students. *Int. J. Bus. Soc. Sci.* **2010**, *1*, 110–116.

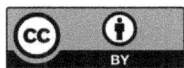

Article

Salivary Oxytocin Concentration Changes during a Group Drumming Intervention for Maltreated School Children

Teruko Yuhi [1,*] , Hiroaki Kyuta [2], Hisa-aki Mori [2], Chihiro Murakami [2], Kazumi Furuhara [1], Mari Okuno [1], Masaki Takahashi [2], Daikei Fuji [2] and Haruhiro Higashida [1]

[1] Department of Basic Research on Social Recognition, Research Center for Child Mental Development, Kanazawa University, Kanazawa 920-8640, Japan; furururukz.999@gmail.com (K.F.); brainsci@med.kanazawa-u.ac.jp (M.O.); haruhiro@med.kanazawa-u.ac.jp (H.H.)
[2] Lumbini Gakuen Ayabe, A Short-Term Therapeutic Institution for Emotionally Disturbed Children, Social Welfare Juridical Corporation Lumbini-en, Ayabe, Kyoto 629-1244, Japan; kyuuta.hiroaki@rouge.plala.or.jp (H.K.); hkty.08450888@gmail.com (H.M.); muracami814@yahoo.co.jp (C.M.); ize00157@nifty.com (M.T.); daikei.fuji@gmail.com (D.F.)
* Correspondence: y-teruko@med.kanazawa-u.ac.jp; Tel.: +81-076-265-2457

Received: 25 July 2017; Accepted: 13 November 2017; Published: 16 November 2017

Abstract: Many emotionally-disturbed children who have been maltreated and are legally separated from their parents or primary caregivers live in group homes and receive compulsory education. Such institutions provide various special intervention programs. Taiko-ensou, a Japanese style of group drumming, is one such program because playing drums in a group may improve children's emotional well-being. However, evidence for its efficacy has not been well established at the biological level. In this study, we measured salivary levels of oxytocin (OT), a neuropeptide associated with social memory and communication, in three conditions (recital, practice, and free sessions) in four classes of school-aged children. Following the sessions, OT concentrations showed changes in various degrees and directions (no change, increases, or decreases). The mean OT concentration changes after each session increased, ranging from 112% to 165%. Plasma OT concentrations were equally sensitive to drum playing in school-aged boys and girls. However, the difference between practice and free play sessions was only significant among elementary school boys aged 8–12 years. The results suggest that younger boys are most responsive to this type of educational music intervention.

Keywords: child abuse; maltreatment; intervention; drum playing; salivary; oxytocin

1. Introduction

Childhood maltreatment represents the most potent predictor of poor mental health across the lifespan [1–3]. Such adversity increases the risk of a wide range of psychiatric disorders, including reactive attachment disorder (RAD) and autism spectrum disorder (ASD) [4–7]. Children with ASD and RAD experience similar difficulties with social relationships [8–10], but there appears to be a difference in the quality of their social interactions. In most cases it is possible to differentiate between children with ASD and children with RAD via structured observation. The most important difference is that RAD is associated with neglect or maltreatment, whereas ASD usually is not [8,9].

Children who are found to have been maltreated are entrusted to a foster parent or admitted to a children's home, a short-term therapeutic institution for emotionally disturbed children, or a children's self-reliance support facility [11–13]. In Japan, emotionally-disturbed children, including those who have been maltreated, are either admitted to a short-term therapeutic institution or treated as out-patients, and receive consultation and other assistance. Children who are resident in such institutions learn to adapt to social life while living together in groups, and also receive compulsory education [12,13].

It is increasingly recognized that music-making interventions can enhance mental health [14–16]. Among them, drumming has long been a part of traditional healing rituals worldwide, and is increasingly used as a therapeutic strategy [17–19]. The features of group drumming programs are known to facilitate mental health recovery. The findings of previous studies support the concept of "creative practice as mutual recovery", demonstrating that group drumming provides a creative and mutual learning space in which mental health recovery can take place [17,18,20]. These reports indicate a shift away from a pro-inflammatory toward an anti-inflammatory immune profile. Consequently, the psychological benefits of group drumming and the underlying biological effects support its therapeutic potential for mental health [18,20]. Drumming is a complex composite intervention with the potential to modulate specific neuroendocrine and neuroimmune parameters in the opposite direction to that of the classic stress response [20].

Recent studies have suggested that oxytocin (OT) plays a role in social memory and behavior [21–28]. OT has positive effects on social and emotional processes in healthy subjects and some individuals diagnosed with a variety of psychiatric disorders [29–33]. Nasal application of OT in subjects with ASD with or without comorbid intellectual disability has been shown to improve social interactions [34–38].

This study was conducted in a facility where children with mild emotional disturbance live and study together. Most of them are isolated from their parents and primary caregivers, owing to maltreatment and neglect. The institute offers special educational intervention programs, such as group drumming, to improve their emotional well-being. However, the facility does not use any biological measures to monitor the beneficial effects of group drumming. Salivary OT can be measured in human saliva, suggesting that it may be a reliable biomarker [39–46]. Therefore, we examined whether maltreated school-aged children exhibited changes in OT concentrations during educational sessions based on Japanese Taiko group drumming (Supplementary Figure S1) [47]. In this study, we measured salivary OT concentrations in children before and after recital or practice drumming sessions and compared them with those in free play sessions. We also analyzed changes in OT concentrations by classifying participants by sex and age, such as boys in the elementary school (8–12 years old) and junior high school (13–15 years old), or girls in the elementary school. We also measured OT concentrations in the children's drumming instructors.

2. Materials and Methods

2.1. Participants

The study recruited 23 boys and five girls aged 8–15 years as voluntary participants (Table 1). The children had lived for between 0.5 and six years in the short-term therapeutic institution for emotionally-disturbed children, run by the Social Welfare Juridical Corporation Lunbini-en (Ayabe, Kyoto, Japan). They attended either the elementary or the junior high school attached to the Lunbini-en. The children were placed in this facility by municipal or prefectural child guidance centers because they were considered to be in need of daily life guidance due to their family environment. We obtained data from three male drumming instructors who taught at the schools (36.2 ± 3 years old).

Table 1. Demographic data.

Standing	Elementary School	Junior High School	Teacher
Age (years)	8–12 (9.9 ± 0.9)	13–15 (14.4 ± 0.4)	33–40 (36.2 ± 3)
Gender			
male	9	13	3
female	5	0	0
Intervention duration (min)			
None	118 ± 16.5 ($n = 6$)		
Practice	108 ± 10.2 ($n = 5$)		
Recital	14.1 ± 3.5 ($n = 12$)		

2.2. Ethics Statement

The study was approved as a non-invasive medical study by the institutional review board of the Social Welfare Juridical Corporation Lunbini-en in 2014 and by Kanazawa University Graduate School of Medicine in 2015 (approval number #2012-1). The study was performed according to the Declaration of Helsinki and the Ethical Guidelines for Clinical Studies of the Ministry of Health, Labor and Welfare of Japan. After they had been given a complete explanation of the study, all of the participants and their caregivers or the child welfare officers in the child guidance centers provided written informed consent. The participants were told that they could choose not to supply their saliva on each occasion, even after agreeing to participate in the study.

2.3. Assessment

The children's salivary OT levels were assessed during 19 sessions of group Taiko drumming (Supplementary Figure S1) from July 2015 to December 2016. The children played freely for the first 10 min. Saliva was collected in a sterile 15-mL polyproprylene tube (Greiner Bio-one Co. Ltd., Tokyo, Japan). Two to five minutes after rinsing with water, the children's mouths filled with newly-secreted saliva. They bit the tube in their mouths and secreted saliva directly into the tube by chewing for 2–4 min. This method was less stressful for such children than using a cotton swab and they were able to complete it by themselves without teachers' assistance. Then they participated in a 5–60 min (14.1 ± 3.5 min, $n = 14$) during recitals on stages in front of an audience (Supplementary Figure S2), or six 80–155 min (108 ± 10.2 min, $n = 6$) practice sessions in a hall at the Lunbini-en (Supplementary Figure S3, upper panels). Saliva was collected a second time after 10 min of all sessions. As a control, saliva was collected 10 min before and after the free play sessions (during which they usually moved, chatted, and read freely) for 90–200 min (118 ± 16.5, $n = 6$) in the same hall or playground of the Lunbini-en (Supplementary Figure S3, lower panels).

2.4. Saliva Collection and Analysis

The saliva samples (0.3–0.8 mL) were collected in polyproprylene tubes and were immediately frozen in dry ice and stored at −20 °C, as described previously [48]. Three days later, they were thawed and centrifuged twice at 4 °C at $1500\times g$ for 15 min. The samples were divided into 1.5-mL microtubes, each containing 100 μL, and kept again at −80 °C until assay.

Salivary OT was measured using a 96-plate commercial OT-ELISA kit (Enzo Life Sciences, Farmingdale, NY, USA), as described previously [48,49]. Measurements were performed in duplicate. Samples (100 μL) without fractionation were treated according to the manufacturer's instructions. The optical density of the samples and standards was measured at wavelengths of 405 and 590 nm by a microplate reader (Bio-Rad, Richmond, CA, USA). Sample concentrations were calculated by MatLab-7 (MathWorks, Inc., Natick, MA, USA) according to the relevant standard curve.

2.5. Statistical Analysis

Two-tailed Student's t tests were used for single comparisons between two groups. One- or two-way analyses of variance were used for data with two or three components, respectively. Post hoc comparisons were performed only when the main effect was statistically significant. The p-values of the multiple comparisons were adjusted using Bonferroni's correction. All data from in vivo and in vitro studies are shown as means ± s.e.m. In all analyses, $p < 0.05$ was taken to indicate statistical significance. All of the analyses were performed using STATA data analysis and statistical software (Stata Corp. LP, College Station, TX, USA).

3. Results

Table 1 shows the demographic characteristics of the participants in the traditional Japanese Taiko group. A total of 23 boys and five girls from the elementary and junior high schools were involved in the sessions, during which three male teachers instructed them to play a piece of music.

The OT concentrations in the saliva collected from the children and adults before the performance and control sessions were determined and used as the baseline OT levels (Table 2). The average baseline salivary OT level did not differ significantly between assessments for any of the groups, but the highest value was obtained from the elementary school boys. The OT concentrations in the saliva after different activities (recital, practice (lesson), and free) were plotted separately for the elementary school boys (Figure 1), junior high school boys (Figure 2), elementary school girls (Figure 3), and teachers (Figure 4). No significant differences were observed before and after sessions in the four groups of participants, except for teachers at the recitals ($p < 0.01$).

Table 2. Baseline concentrations of oxytocin (pg/mL).

	Boys		Girls	Adults	
	Elementary School	**Junior High School**	**Elementary School**	**Teachers**	
Free activity	166 ± 34 (32)	259 ± 23 (39)	179 ± 30 (26)	142 ± 34 (14)	$F_{3,109} = 3.36$ ($p = 0.0215$)
Practice	83 ± 29 (14)	176 ± 48 (16)	123 ± 22 (13)	103 ± 21 (8)	$F_{3,45} = 1.61$ ($p = 0.1992$)
Recital	149 ± 21 (44)	265 ± 31* # (63)	186 ± 20 (34)	138 ± 14 (33)	$F_{3,173} = 6.09$ ($p = 0.0006$)
	$F_{2,84} = 1.01$ ($p = 0.3681$)	$F_{2,122} = 1.76$ ($p = 0.1768$)	$F_{2,70} = 1.23$ ($p = 0.2989$)	$F_{2,58} = 0.01$ ($p = 0.9884$)	

One-way ANOVA analysis of each matrics is shown. * # $p < 0.01$ for recital in elementary school boys and teachers (Bonferroni's test).

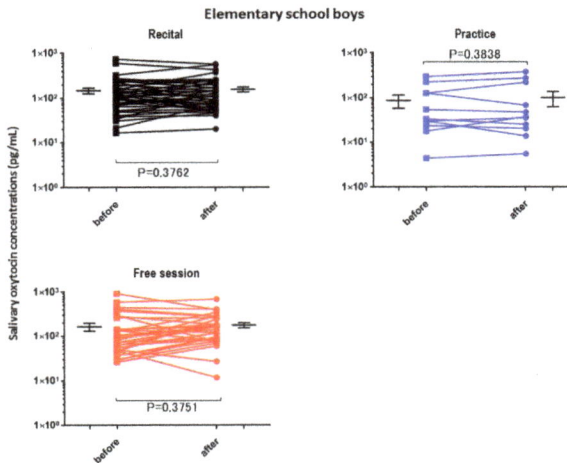

Figure 1. Changes in elementary school boys' oxytocin levels before and after a single play session. Oxytocin levels are for the first (before) and second (after) salivary samples. Saliva was collected at each recital ($n = 52$), practice ($n = 11$), and free play ($n = 33$) session. p values are for two-tailed Student's t-tests.

The difference of salivary OT concentrations before and after the activity was calculated. Since the conditions differed in terms of whether an instrument was played and the duration, we compared the changes in OT between non-obligatory activities and practice with the instrument with a similar time gap (Figure 5). Similarly, the difference was compared between recital and practice, both of which involved playing the drums (Figure 6). Significant changes in the ratio of salivary OT levels before and after activities and between playing practice and free sessions were observed only in the elementary school boys (two-way Student's *t*-test, $n = 11$–34, $p < 0.02$).

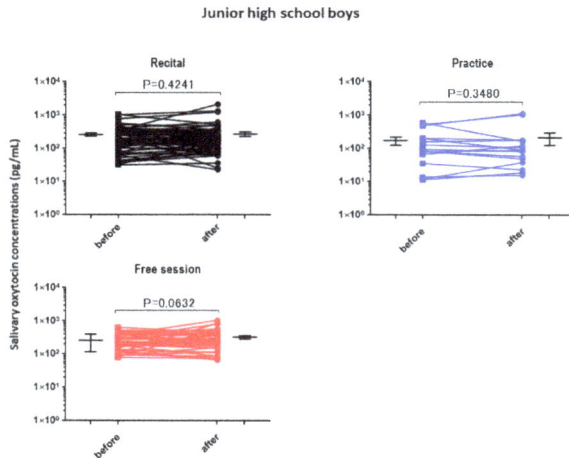

Figure 2. Changes in junior high school boys' oxytocin levels before and after a single play session. Oxytocin levels are for the first (before) and second (after) salivary samples. Saliva was collected at each recital ($n = 61$), practice ($n = 17$), and free play ($n = 55$) session. *p* values are for two-tailed Student's *t*-tests.

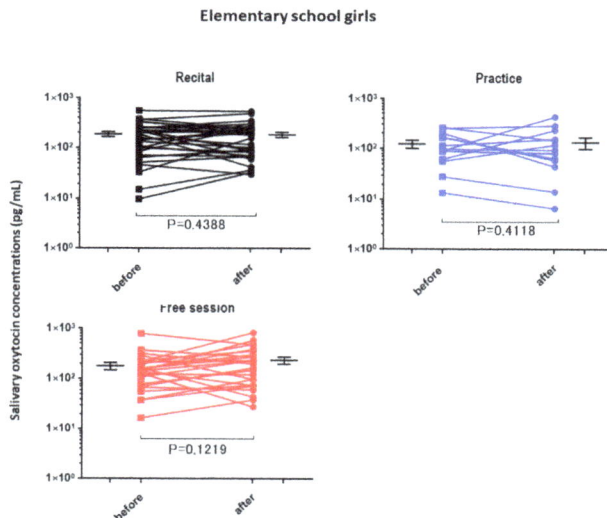

Figure 3. Changes in elementary school girls' oxytocin levels before and after a single play session. Oxytocin levels are for the first (before) and second (after) salivary samples. Saliva was collected at each recital ($n = 33$), practice ($n = 14$), and free play ($n = 30$) session. *p* values are for two-tailed Student's *t*-tests. A significant difference was found for the recital session.

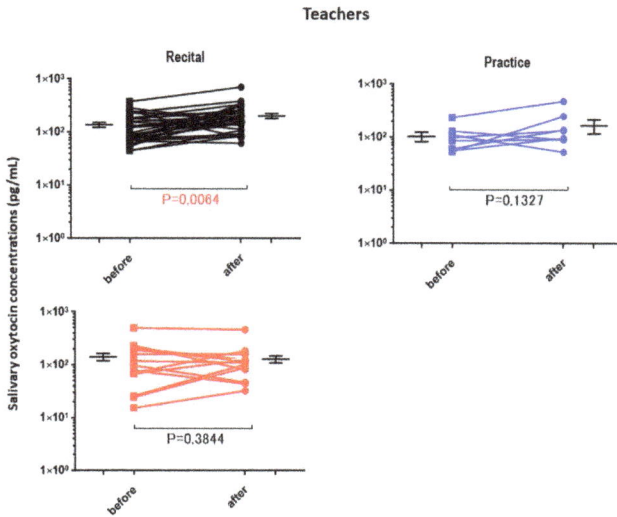

Figure 4. Changes in teachers' oxytocin levels before and after a single play session. Oxytocin levels are for the first (before) and second (after) salivary samples. Saliva was collected at each recital (*n* = 33), practice (*n* = 8), and free play (*n* = 14) session. *p* values are for two-tailed Student's *t*-tests.

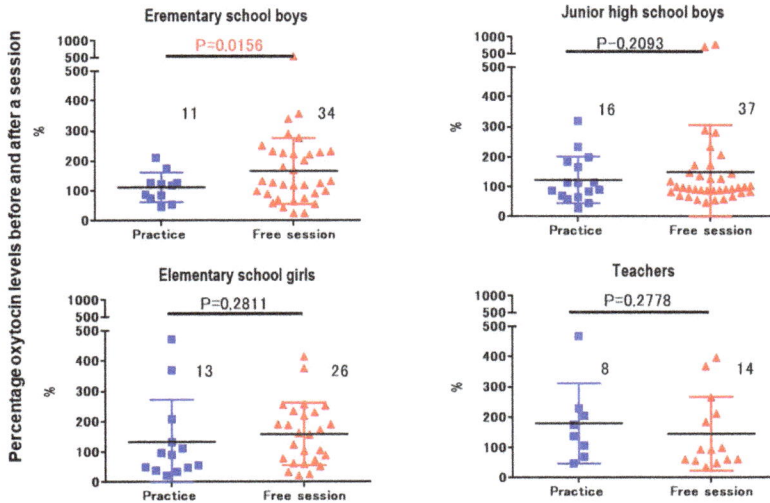

Figure 5. Changes in oxytocin levels before and after a single session. Percentage of oxytocin levels for the first (before) saliva over the second (after) saliva samples. Saliva was collected at practice and free play sessions from elementary school boys, junior high school boys, elementary school girls, and teachers. *p* values are for two-tailed Student's *t*-tests.

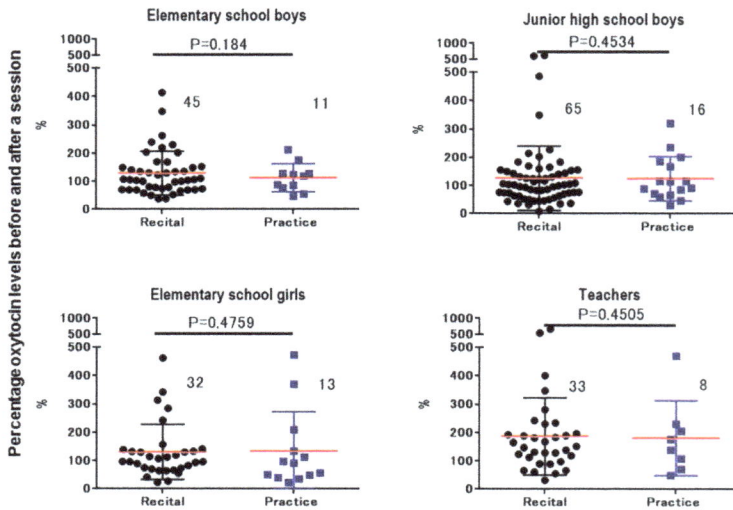

Figure 6. Changes in oxytocin levels before and after a single session. Percentage of oxytocin levels for the first (before) saliva over the second (after) saliva samples. Saliva was collected at recital and practice sessions from elementary school boys, junior high school boys, elementary school girls, and teachers. *p* values are for two-tailed Student's *t*-tests.

4. Discussion

We examined the biological effects of playing music in a Japanese Taiko drumming group. This activity was performed less than once a week as part of an educational intervention for children living and studying in a short-term therapeutic institution for emotionally disturbed children, most of whom were legally separated from their parents or caregivers because of maltreatment [12,13]. The results indicated that the children's mean salivary OT concentrations were increased to various degrees after the activity sessions. The smallest increase was observed in the elementary school boys during the practice session and the largest change was in the girls of the elementary school after the free session. However, the only significant difference was between practice and free sessions for boys aged 8–12 years (Figure 5), although a similar tendency was observed in the junior high school boys and elementary school girls, it was not significant. The change in OT concentration was in the reverse direction, i.e., higher during practice than free time, although in the teachers' case it was during drumming instruction.

The reason such significant changes were observed only in younger boys may be that drum playing creates a better atmosphere for younger boys than older ones. In other words, drum playing may not be stressful for older boys but for younger boys because high school boys are already familiar with drumming. Drumming on a stage in front of an audience (recital) and playing for practice (rehearsal) may be essentially different for the players. In addition, the performing time was also different: recitals lasted only 14 min on average, compared with 108 min for practice. This makes it difficult to compare the three groups on the different conditions, but as the experiment did not interfere with the institutional routine, optimal ecological validity was maintained.

However, even shorter activities seemed to be stressful. The average OT concentrations were lower after group drumming recital and practice sessions than before. The effects were evident in boys, and seemed to be due to the group drumming rather than playing individually, which created some stress. The OT concentration changes before and after free play, as a control condition, were in the opposite direction.

In relation to our study, there are several interesting reports on playing music as a group, which describe differences between singing alone (solo) and in a group. Schladt et al. [50] reported that OT increased in the case of solo singing but not in choir. This suggests that, although singing in a group seems to be a joyful experience and one that facilitates bonding [51], it can be rather stressful. Singing lessons for professional or amateur singers are not the same, because professional singers are achievement-oriented, but amateurs sing for self-actualization or self-expression [52]. For the school children in the current study, it is likely that OT increased owing to the release of emotional tension in the recital or practice sessions. In the teachers, OT significantly increased in the recital sessions (Figure 4), probably because they were satisfied by the children's successful performance.

Overall behavior while staying in this therapeutic institution generally improved: the children thought that the Lumbini-en is safe and secure, solved vigilance, and opened their hearts to the surroundings. They became to sleep well, to feel less anxiety, and less likely to panic with a trivial chance. They became to control themselves according to their opponents and situations. They participated in group activities and continued to go to the inside school. They tried to decide their own lives by themselves, grew self-confidence, and finally got to have the hope of going to alive. Such outcomes of individuals were assessed using the school's behavior and study records. Child welfare officers and teachers rated the children's behavior using a questionnaire. In addition, the officers and teachers felt that drumming can be a positive and effective educational intervention to improve children's behavior.

Next, we considered the relationship between OT concentrations and individual's behaviors. Participants were classified according to the initial OT levels and changes in OT levels before and after a single session. The drumming teachers reported that individuals in the group with OT levels in the recital and free sessions that were higher than average are restless, weaker to stimulation, autistic and hyperactive, compared with other individuals (Supplementary Figure S4). In the teacher's records, participants who showed higher rates of change in OT levels before and after recital or free sessions are relatively hyperactive compared with individuals in other classes (Supplementary Figure S5). These results, interestingly, indicate that OT levels modified to a greater extent in a category of hyperactive boys and girls.

It is worth considering the well-known correlation between OT and group cohesion. It is interesting that in boys free play tended to lead to increased OT levels than did practical lessons. This may be due to the cohesiveness effect. To perform in a recital is stressful, particularly for children with disturbed social function, and is likely to reduce vagal activity and cohesiveness. Increases in OT concentrations correspond to increased vagal activity and vice versa, resulting from the brain mechanism as described in prairie voles [53]. In line with this, a study by Harmat and Theorell [54] showed dramatically reduced vagal activity during a concert compared with during a rehearsal, and particularly among those musicians who reported nervousness in recital.

This study had some limitations. Although the measures of salivary OT were taken two years apart, the number of school children involved was small. Opportunity sampling meant that the number of participants was not constant on each occasion.

It has been reported that salivary OT is frequently measured as the biomarker [41,43,55–58], however, though some of the saliva components interact with the labeled OT in the assay mixture [59]. To test this, we first measured samples spiked with 50, 100, 200, and 400 pg/mL. Even the very high level was observed with no addition of spiked OT, suggesting an interaction with nonspecific antibody-interacting substances. Even with interacting substances in the samples, the EIA monitored concentrations were proportional to the spiked OT concentrations, suggesting that monitored values are useful for calculating the ratio between values. Therefore, the difference of OT concentrations before and after the sessions shown in Figures 5 and 6 seems to be reliable.

This study did not address behavioral changes in the children at school. Such tests should be performed using a standard questionnaire survey and the children's school records. Teachers in the Institution have the impression that drumming improves the behavior of children living in care.

In general, they report that the caregiver-teacher-child relationship improves within the first month up to the end of the year.

In conclusion, this study found that maltreated children responded reasonably well and benefitted from a group drumming intervention, as indicated by their increased salivary OT concentrations. The intervention was effective because the children experienced stress, and the stress-relax cycle is linked to the capacity to control emotional reaction.

Supplementary Materials: The following are available online at http://www.mdpi.com/2076-3425/7/11/152/s1; Figure S1: Various types of Wataiko (Japanese percussions) used for music intervention in group, Figure S2: Recitals performed in front of audiences in various stages in wearing with a festival uniform, Figure S3: Upper panels, practice in a hall; lower panels: free sessions, Figure S4: Oxytocin concentrations of individuals before recital and free play sessions, Figure S5: Changes in oxytocin concentrations of individuals before and after recital and free play sessions.

Acknowledgments: This work was supported by the industry-Academia Collaborative R and D Programs (COI) grant-in-aid from the Ministry of Education, Culture, Sports, Science and Technology of Japan. We thank Maki Rooksby for critical reading. We thank Rachel Baron, from Edanz Group (www.edanzediting.com/ac) for editing a draft of this manuscript. Funding: The industry-Academia Collaborative Research and Development Programs (COI) by the Ministry of Education, Culture, Sports, Science and Technology of Japan (MEXT).

Author Contributions: H.H., M.T. and D.F. designed the experiments. H.H. and T.Y. wrote the manuscript. H.K., H.-a.M., C.M., K.F., M.O., M.T. and T.Y. performed the experiments.

Conflicts of Interest: The authors declare no conflict of interest.

References

1. Teicher, M.H.; Tomoda, A.; Andersen, S.L. Neurobiological consequences of early stress and childhood maltreatment: Are results from human and animal studies comparable? *Ann. N. Y. Acad. Sci.* **2006**, *1071*, 313–323. [CrossRef] [PubMed]
2. McCrory, E.J.; Viding, E. The theory of latent vulnerability: Reconceptualizing the link between childhood maltreatment and psychiatric disorder. *Dev. Psychopathol.* **2015**, *27*, 493–505. [CrossRef] [PubMed]
3. McCrory, E.J.; Gerin, M.I.; Viding, E. Annual Research Review: Childhood maltreatment, latent vulnerability and the shift to preventative psychiatry—The contribution of functional brain imaging. *J. Child Psychol. Psychiatry* **2017**, *58*, 338–357. [CrossRef] [PubMed]
4. Jaffee, S.R. Child maltreatment and risk for psychopathology in childhood and adulthood. *Annu. Rev. Clin. Psychol.* **2017**, *13*, 525–551. [CrossRef] [PubMed]
5. Busso, D.S.; McLaughlin, K.A.; Brueck, S.; Peverill, M.; Gold, A.L.; Sheridan, M.A. Child Abuse, Neural Structure, and Adolescent Psychopathology: A Longitudinal Study. *J. Am. Acad. Child Adolesc. Psychiatry* **2017**, *56*, 321–328. [CrossRef] [PubMed]
6. Stein, M.B.; Campbell-Sills, L.; Ursano, R.J.; Rosellini, A.J.; Colpe, L.J.; He, F.; Heeringa, S.G.; Nock, M.K.; Sampson, N.A.; Schoenbaum, M.; et al. Childhood Maltreatment and Lifetime Suicidal Behaviors Among New Soldiers in the US Army: Results From the Army Study to Assess Risk and Resilience in Service members (Army STARRS). *J. Clin. Psychiatry* **2017**. [CrossRef] [PubMed]
7. Oshio, T.; Umeda, M. Gender-specific linkages of parents' childhood physical abuse and neglect with children's problem behaviour: Evidence from Japan. *BMC Public Health* **2016**, *14*, 403. [CrossRef] [PubMed]
8. Mayes, S.D.; Calhoun, S.L.; Waschbusch, D.A.; Baweja, R. Autism and reactive attachment/disinhibited social engagement disorders: Co-occurrence and differentiation. *Clin. Child Psychol. Psychiatry* **2016**, *22*, 620–631. [CrossRef] [PubMed]
9. Davidson, C.; O'Hare, A.; Mactaggart, F.; Green, J.; Young, D.; Gillberg, C.; Minnis, H. Social relationship difficulties in autism and reactive attachment disorder: Improving diagnostic validity through structured assessment. *Res. Dev. Disabil.* **2015**, *40*, 63–72. [CrossRef] [PubMed]
10. McLaughlin, K.A.; Greif Green, J.; Gruber, M.J.; Sampson, N.A.; Zaslavsky, A.M.; Kessler, R.C. Childhood adversities and first onset of psychiatric disorders in a national sample of US adolescents. *Arch. Gen. Psychiatry* **2012**, *69*, 1151–1160. [CrossRef] [PubMed]
11. Hermenau, K.; Kaltenbach, E.; Mkinga, G.; Hecker, T. Improving care quality and preventing maltreatment in institutional care—A feasibility study with caregivers. *Front. Psychol.* **2015**, *14*, 937. [CrossRef] [PubMed]

12. Matsushige, T.; Tsutsui, T.; Ogata, M. Mutual aid' beyond formal institutions: Integrated home care in Japan. *Curr. Sociol.* **2012**, *60*, 538–550. [CrossRef]

13. Tsutsui, T.; Otaga, M.; Higashino, S.; Cottencin, A. Effects of presence in prefectures of short-term therapeutic institutions for emotionally disturbed children on the types of children that have to be taken care of in self-reliance support facilities and foster homes. *J. Natl. Inst. Public Health* **2013**, *62*, 204–212.

14. Daykin, N.; de Viggiani, N.; Pilkington, P.; Moriarty, Y. Music making for health, well-being and behaviour change in youth justice settings: A systematic review. *Health Promot. Int.* **2013**, *28*, 197–210. [CrossRef] [PubMed]

15. Cevasco, A.M. Effects of the therapist's nonverbal behavior on participation and affect of individuals with Alzheimer's disease during group music therapy sessions. *Music Ther.* **2010**, *47*, 282–299. [CrossRef]

16. Altenmüller, E.; Schlaug, G. Apollo's gift: New aspects of neurologic music therapy. *Prog. Brain Res.* **2015**, *217*, 237–252. [PubMed]

17. Perkins, R.; Ascenso, S.; Atkins, L.; Fancourt, D.; Williamon, A. Making music for mental health: How group drumming mediates recovery. *Psychol. Well Being* **2016**, *6*, 11. [CrossRef] [PubMed]

18. Fancourt, D.; Perkins, R.; Ascenso, S.; Carvalho, L.A.; Steptoe, A.; Williamon, A. Effects of Group Drumming Interventions on Anxiety, Depression, Social Resilience and Inflammatory Immune Response among Mental Health Service Users. *PLoS ONE* **2016**, *11*, e0151136. [CrossRef] [PubMed]

19. Ho, P.; Tsao, J.C.; Bloch, L.; Zeltzer, L.K. The impact of group drumming on social-emotional behavior in low-income children. *Evid. Based Complement. Altern. Med.* **2011**, *2011*, 250708. [CrossRef] [PubMed]

20. Bittman, B.B.; Berk, L.S.; Felten, D.L.; Westengard, J.; Simonton, O.C.; Pappas, J.; Ninehouser, M. Composite effects of group drumming music therapy on modulation of neuroendocrine-immune parameters in normal subjects. *Altern. Ther. Health Med.* **2001**, *7*, 38–47. [PubMed]

21. Kosfeld, M.; Heinrichs, M.; Zak, P.J.; Fischbacher, U.; Fehr, E. Oxytocin increases trust in humans. *Nature* **2005**, *35*, 673–676. [CrossRef] [PubMed]

22. Jin, D.; Liu, H.X.; Hirai, H.; Torashima, T.; Nagai, T.; Lopatina, O.; Shnayder, N.A.; Yamada, K.; Noda, M.; Seike, T.; et al. CD38 is critical for social behaviour by regulating oxytocin secretion. *Nature* **2007**, *446*, 41–45. [CrossRef] [PubMed]

23. Feldman, R.; Monakhov, M.; Pratt, M.; Ebstein, R.P. Oxytocin Pathway Genes: Evolutionary Ancient System Impacting on Human Affiliation, Sociality, and Psychopathology. *Biol. Psychiatry* **2016**, *79*, 174–184. [CrossRef] [PubMed]

24. Insel, T.R. The challenge of translation in social neuroscience: A review of oxytocin, vasopressin, and affiliative behavior. *Neuron* **2010**, *65*, 768–779. [CrossRef] [PubMed]

25. Higashida, H.; Yokoyama, S.; Huang, J.J.; Liu, L.; Ma, W.J.; Akther, S.; Higashida, C.; Kikuchi, M.; Minabe, Y.; Munesue, T. Social memory, amnesia, and autism: Brain oxytocin secretion is regulated by NAD+ metabolites and single nucleotide polymorphisms of CD38. *Neurochem. Int.* **2012**, *61*, 828–838. [CrossRef] [PubMed]

26. Dulac, C.; O'Connell, L.A.; Wu, Z. Neural control of maternal and paternal behaviors. *Science* **2014**, *345*, 765–770. [CrossRef] [PubMed]

27. Neumann, I.D.; Landgraf, R. Balance of brain oxytocin and vasopressin: Implications for anxiety, depression, and social behaviors. *Trends Neurosci.* **2012**, *35*, 649–659. [CrossRef] [PubMed]

28. Burkett, J.P.; Andari, E.; Johnson, Z.V.; Curry, D.C.; de Waal, F.B.; Young, L.J. Oxytocin-dependent consolation behavior in rodents. *Science* **2016**, *351*, 375–378. [CrossRef] [PubMed]

29. Zhang, R.; Xu, X.J.; Zhang, H.F.; Han, S.P.; Han, J.S. The Role of the Oxytocin/Arginine Vasopressin System in Animal Models of Autism Spectrum Disorder. *Adv. Anat. Embryol. Cell Biol.* **2017**, *224*, 135–158. [PubMed]

30. Quintana, D.S.; Dieset, I.; Elvsåshagen, T.; Westlye, L.; Andreassen, O.A. Oxytocin system dysfunction as a common mechanism underlying metabolic syndrome and psychiatric symptoms in schizophrenia and bipolar disorders. *Front. Neuroendocrinol.* **2017**, *45*, 1–10. [CrossRef] [PubMed]

31. MacDonald, K.; Feifel, D. Oxytocin's role in anxiety: A critical appraisal. *Brain Res.* **2014**, *1580*, 2–56. [CrossRef] [PubMed]

32. Munesue, T.; Yokoyama, S.; Nakamura, K.; Anitha, A.; Yamada, K.; Hayashi, K.; Asaka, T.; Liu, H.X.; Jin, D.; Koizumi, K.; et al. Two genetic variants of CD38 in subjects with autism spectrum disorder and controls. *Neurosci. Res.* **2010**, *67*, 181–191. [CrossRef] [PubMed]

33. Romano, A.; Tempesta, B.; Micioni Di Bonaventura, M.V.; Gaetani, S. From Autism to Eating Disorders and More: The Role of Oxytocin in Neuropsychiatric Disorders. *Front. Neurosci.* **2016**, *9*, 497. [CrossRef] [PubMed]

34. Munesue, T.; Nakamura, H.; Kikuchi, M.; Miura, Y.; Takeuch, N.; Anme, T.; Nanba, E.; Adachi, K.; Tsubouchi, K.; Sai, Y.; et al. Oxytocin for Male Subjects with Autism Spectrum Disorder and Comorbid Intellectual Disabilities: A Randomized Pilot Study. *Front. Psychiatry* **2016**, *7*, 2. [CrossRef] [PubMed]

35. Kosaka, H.; Okamoto, Y.; Munesue, T.; Yamasue, H.; Inohara, K.; Fujioka, T.; Anme, T.; Orisaka, M.; Ishitobi, M.; Jung, M.; et al. Oxytocin efficacy is modulated by dosage and oxytocin receptor genotype in young adults with high-functioning autism: A 24-week randomized clinical trial. *Transl. Psychiatry* **2016**, *6*, e872. [CrossRef] [PubMed]

36. Watanabe, T.; Kuroda, M.; Kuwabara, H.; Aoki, Y.; Iwashiro, N.; Tatsunobu, N.; Takao, H.; Nippashi, Y.; Kawakubo, Y.; Kunimatsu, A.; et al. Clinical and neural effects of six-week administration of oxytocin on core symptoms of autism. *Brain* **2015**, *138*, 3400–3412. [CrossRef] [PubMed]

37. Yatawara, C.J.; Einfeld, S.L.; Hickie, I.B.; Davenport, T.A.; Guastella, A.J. The effect of oxytocin nasal spray on social interaction deficits observed in young children with autism: A randomized clinical crossover trial. *Mol. Psychiatry* **2016**, *21*, 1225–1231. [CrossRef] [PubMed]

38. Guastella, A.J.; Gray, K.M.; Rinehart, N.J.; Alvares, G.A.; Tonge, B.J.; Hickie, I.B.; Keating, C.M.; Cacciotti-Saija, C.; Einfeld, S.L. The effects of a course of intranasal oxytocin on social behaviors in youth diagnosed with autism spectrum disorders: A randomized controlled trial. *J. Child Psychol. Psychiatry* **2015**, *56*, 444–452. [CrossRef] [PubMed]

39. Carter, C.S.; Pournajafi-Nazarloo, H.; Kramer, K.M.; Ziegler, T.E.; White-Traut, R.; Bello, D.; Schwertz, D. Oxytocin: Behavioral associations and potential as a salivary biomarker. *Ann. N. Y. Acad. Sci.* **2007**, *1098*, 312–322. [CrossRef] [PubMed]

40. Van Ijzendoorn, M.H.; Bhandari, R.; van der Veen, R.; Grewen, K.M.; Bakermans-Kranenburg, M.J. Elevated salivary levels of oxytocin persist more than 7 h after intranasal administration. *Front. Neurosci.* **2012**, *6*, 174. [CrossRef] [PubMed]

41. Huffmeijer, R.; Alink, L.R.; Tops, M.; Grewen, K.M.; Light, K.C.; Bakermans-Kranenburg, M.J.; Ijzendoorn, M.H. Salivary levels of oxytocin remain elevated for more than two hours after intranasal oxytocin administration. *Neuro Endocrinol. Lett.* **2012**, *33*, 21–25. [PubMed]

42. Weisman, O.; Schneiderman, I.; Zagoory-Sharon, O.; Feldman, R. Salivary vasopressin increases following intranasal oxytocin administration. *Peptides* **2013**, *40*, 99–103. [CrossRef] [PubMed]

43. Bhandari, R.; Bakermans-Kranenburg, M.J.; van der Veen, R.; Parsons, C.E.; Young, K.S.; Grewen, K.M.; Stein, A.; Kringelbach, M.L.; van IJzendoorn, M.H. Salivary oxytocin mediates the association between emotional maltreatment and responses to emotional infant faces. *Physiol. Behav.* **2014**, *131*, 123–128. [CrossRef] [PubMed]

44. Fujisawa, T.X.; Tanaka, S.; Saito, D.N.; Kosaka, H.; Tomoda, A. Visual attention for social information and salivary oxytocin levels in preschool children with autism spectrum disorders: An eye-tracking study. *Front. Neurosci.* **2014**, *8*, 295. [CrossRef] [PubMed]

45. Koven, N.S.; Max, L.K. Basal salivary oxytocin level predicts extra- but not intra-personal dimensions of emotional intelligence. *Psychoneuroendocrinology* **2014**, *44*, 20–29. [CrossRef] [PubMed]

46. Jong, T.R.; Menon, R.; Bludau, A.; Grund, T.; Biermeier, V.; Klampfl, S.M.; Jurek, B.; Bosch, O.J.; Hellhammer, J.; Neumann, I.D. Salivary oxytocin concentrations in response to running, sexual self-stimulation, breastfeeding and the TSST: The Regensburg Oxytocin Challenge (ROC) study. *Psychoneuroendocrinology* **2015**, *62*, 381–388. [CrossRef] [PubMed]

47. Mizuno, E.; Sakuma, H. Wadaiko performance enhances synchronized motion of mentally disabled persons. *Percept. Mot. Skills* **2013**, *116*, 187–196. [CrossRef] [PubMed]

48. Tsuji, S.; Yuhi, T.; Furuhara, K.; Ohta, S.; Shimizu, Y.; Higashida, H. Salivary oxytocin concentrations in seven boys with autism spectrum disorder received massage from their mothers: A pilot study. *Front. Psychiatry* **2015**, *21*, 58. [CrossRef] [PubMed]

49. MacLean, E.L.; Gesquiere, L.R.; Gee, N.; Levy, K.; Martin, W.L.; Carter, C.S. Validation of salivary oxytocin and vasopressin as biomarkers in domestic dogs. *J. Neurosci. Methods* **2017**, *293*, 67–76. [CrossRef] [PubMed]

50. Schladt, T.M.; Nordmann, G.C.; Emilius, R.; Kudielka, B.M.; de Jong, T.R.; Neumann, I.D. Choir versus Solo Singing: Effects on Mood, and Salivary Oxytocin and Cortisol Concentrations. *Front. Hum. Neurosci.* **2017**, *11*, 430. [CrossRef] [PubMed]

51. Kreutz, G. Does singing facilitate social bonding? *Music Med.* **2014**, *6*, 51–60.

52. Grape, C.; Sandgren, M.; Hansson, L.-O.; Ericson, M.; Theorell, T. Does singing promote well-being? An empirical study of professional and amateur singers during a singing lesson. *Integr. Physiol. Behav. Sci.* **2003**, *38*, 65–74. [CrossRef] [PubMed]

53. Yee, J.R.; Kenkel, W.M.; Frijling, J.L.; Dodhia, S.; Onishi, K.G.; Tovar, S.; Saber, M.J.; Lewis, G.F.; Liu, W.; Porges, S.W.; et al. Oxytocin promotes functional coupling between paraventricular nucleus and both sympathetic and parasympathetic cardioregulatory nuclei. *Horm. Behav.* **2016**, *80*, 82–91. [CrossRef] [PubMed]

54. Harmat, L.; Theorell, T. Heart rate variability during singing and flute playing. *Music Med.* **2010**, *2*, 10–17. [CrossRef]

55. Javor, A.; Riedl, R.; Kindermann, H.; Brandstätter, W.; Ransmayr, G.; Gabriel, M. Correlation of plasma and salivary oxytocin in healthy young men—Experimental evidence. *Neuro Endocrinol. Lett.* **2014**, *35*, 470–473. [PubMed]

56. Kanat, M.; Heinrichs, M.; Domes, G. Oxytocin and the social brain: Neural mechanisms and perspectives in human research. *Brain Res.* **2014**, *1580*, 160–171. [CrossRef] [PubMed]

57. Carson, D.S.; Berquist, S.W.; Trujillo, T.H.; Garner, J.P.; Hannah, S.L.; Hyde, S.A.; Sumiyoshi, R.D.; Jackson, L.P.; Moss, J.K.; Strehlow, M.C.; et al. Cerebrospinal fluid and plasma oxytocin concentrations are positively correlated and negatively predict anxiety in children. *Mol. Psychiatry* **2015**, *20*, 1085–1090. [CrossRef] [PubMed]

58. Nishizato, M.; Fujisawa, T.X.; Kosaka, H.; Tomoda, A. Developmental changes in social attention and oxytocin levels in infants and children. *Sci. Rep.* **2017**, *7*, 2540. [CrossRef] [PubMed]

59. Leng, G.; Sabatier, N. Measuring Oxytocin and Vasopressin: Bioassays, Immunoassays and Random Numbers. *J. Neuroendocrinol.* **2016**, *28*. [CrossRef] [PubMed]

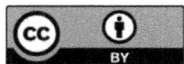

MDPI AG
St. Alban-Anlage 66
4052 Basel
Switzerland
Tel. +41 61 683 77 34
Fax +41 61 302 89 18
www.mdpi.com

Brain Sciences Editorial Office
E-mail: brainsciences@mdpi.com
www.mdpi.com/journal/brainsciences

www.ingramcontent.com/pod-product-compliance
Lightning Source LLC
Chambersburg PA
CBHW051909210326
41597CB00033B/6089